I AM

Aspien *Woman*

The Unique Characteristics, Traits and Gifts of Adult Females on the Autism Spectrum

By

Tania A. Marshall

I am AspienWoman: The Unique Characteristics, Traits, and Gifts of Adult Females on the Autism Spectrum.

Disclaimer
All the information, techniques, skills and concepts contained within this publication are of the nature of general comment only, and are not in any way recommended as individual advice. The intent is to offer a variety of information to provide a wider range of choices now and in the future, recognising that we all have widely diverse circumstances and viewpoints. Should any reader choose to make use of the information contained herein, this is their decision, and the author and publisher do not assume any responsibilities whatsoever under any conditions or circumstances. The author and publisher does not take responsibility for the results of the reader's decision to use this information. It is recommended that the reader obtain their own independent advice.

AspienWoman has no responsibility for the persistence or accuracy of URLs for external or third-party internet websites referred to in this publication, and does not guarantee that any content on such websites is, or will remain, accurate or appropriate.

***Models are for illustrative purposes only, unless clearly stated otherwise.

***All quotes are used with clear and expressed consent from the participant.

Table of Contents

Dedication..9

Introduction 10

Acknowledgements 13

Testimonials...15

Foreword 20

Poem Deer by Aniko, Hungary 22

Psychedelic Chameleon, written by Rachel Phillips, United Kingdom....23

Who am I? 25

Cognitive Style/Personality Type..37

Subtypes 51

Social..65

Education/Work...75

Sensory Sensitivities 93

Emotional...109

Communication/Language 121

Common Interests 132

Gender, Family and Relationships 148

Strengths..158

Challenges 170

Stages Leading up to an Adult Diagnosis.................................184

Important AspienWoman Needs...197

Real-life AspienWoman Superhero Mentors

Dr Temple Grandin 209

Professor Katherine Milla 212

Lauren Lovejoy 214

Jeanette Purkis 217

Olley Edwards 219

Jen Saunders 221

Chou Chou Scantlin 223

Laura Golden 225

Chelsea Hopkins-Allan 227

Maja Toudal 230

Elisabeth Wiklander 232

April Griffin 236

Marguerite (Margo) Comeau 238

Annette Harkness 241

Megan Barnes 243

Samantha Craft 246

Genevieve Kingston 248

Brandy Nightingale 249

Shan Ellis Williams 251

Sybelle Silverphoenix 252

Dena Gassner 255

Xolie Morra Cogley 257

Jessica Ivey 259

Lexington Sherbin 261

Appendix 1 263
Commonly observed characteristics, traits and strengths of adult females

Appendix 2 277
Ideas for using I Am AspienWoman

Appendix 3 279
My Unique Strengths List

Appendix 4 282
20 Reasons to Obtain an Adult Formal Diagnosis

Disclosure 284

References 285

Highly Recommended Resources 289

Further Projects 291

Future Titles 296

Author's Books 298

About the Author 299

Notes 301

In Loving Memory of my Father

This book is dedicated to the 24 mentors in this book and the many AspienWomen around the world who, like warriors and superheroes, strive tenaciously with their unique and extraordinary gifts and challenges.

Introduction

I Am: Two of the most powerful words, for what you put after them shapes your reality.

AspienGirl® : \as-pee-en-ger-l\; AspienWoman :\aspee-en-wo-man\

1. a young female with Autism or Asperger Syndrome
2. an adult female with Autism or Asperger Syndrome
3. a female with a differently wired brain
4. a positive strengths-based perspective and identity designed to support and assist females on the spectrum and help them discover themselves, their unique abilities and strengths; to showcase value, ability and contribution; living with both gifts and disability, a focus on strengths, yet not ignoring the challenges

Over the years, I have worked with a large group of females, of all ages, who have a stunning array of gifts and talents, in addition to challenges. This particular group of individuals all have the characteristic traits of Asperger Syndrome or high functioning Autism. Many of them are gifted in a variety of ways. Most have discussed feeling different, alone, from another planet, or era; hence the term Planet Aspien. The use of terms, for example 'AspienWoman', are used affectionately and serve as a strengths-based identity for a group of females who often feel isolated on populous planet Earth.

In researching this book I've also spoken to women from around the world, including Canada, the United States of America, the United Kingdom, the European Union, China, Japan, Singapore, Malaysia, New Zealand, Australia, South Africa, France, Italy, Spain, Germany, Norway, Sweden, Denmark, Scotland, India and Israel.

This book is a conversation starter, a visual illumination of a group of adult females all over the world, all experiencing similar strengths and challenges, in varying degrees. This book is based on professional private practice experience, anecdotal evidence and current research. The women in this book are from the 'lost generation', the generation where Autism did not exist as a diagnosis. Today, many women struggle to obtain a diagnosis and are knocked back because they do not fit the 'male' criteria. This is the current gender bias, with some female research, little to no female assessment tools and no female-based interventions.

What I have learnt is that many of these women are 'warriors' and when supported and provided with the right environmental fit, are able to use their unique combination of gifts and talents to overcome their challenges and limitations, in addition to sharing their gifts with the world. Each day I have witnessed females working in 'superhero' drive, fighting daily battles that even people in their family, at work, university or community are unaware of. Through sheer determination, I have witnessed females picking themselves back up, dusting themselves off and going forward, in a positive and healthy way. That is a warrior. Go forward, warriors, each one of you, knowing you are one of many paving a positive way for the future AspienGirls and AspienWomen who may be just now finding out who they are, regardless of their age.

In the year since its release, I Am Aspiengirl® has gone onto become a best seller, win an Ippy eLit Gold Medal Award and be recognised by ASPECT Autism Australia with a National Recognition Award in the Advancement Category.

I Am AspienGirl® is now available in Spanish with the following languages being completed and/or released within the next year: Italian, German, Japanese, Norwegian, Dutch, Chinese, Brazilian Portuguese, Hebrew and French.

After *I Am AspienGirl®* was released in June 2014, the AspienGirl® team was inundated with emails, stories, messages and letters. Many of them were from females themselves or from their family members, their loved ones and professionals. We received pictures, poetry, art, short and long stories, pleas for help, support and requests for information. We had people, of all ages, wanting to be a part of the Be Your Own Superhero Project (www.aspiengirl.com). We received messages from a number of countries wanting to know more about female Autism, offering their translation skills to assist in getting the information made available in other languages, wanting to know where to go to start the process of an assessment. Messages came in from parents and professionals saying they were using the book to explain the diagnosis or as a reference point for explaining or discussing certain characteristics. Many of the messages or testimonials referred to the format of the book, in particular the use of images and quotes which combined together showcase a particular trait, characteristic or talent, being an effective way to promote awareness and educate others.

I Am AspienWoman is the sequel and based on a blog I wrote two years ago entitled 'Aspienwomen: Moving towards an adult female profile of Autism/Asperger Syndrome'. As we go to press this blog has been viewed approximately 225,000 times in two years and has been translated into a variety of languages, reblogged and cited in a variety of publications.

Women with Autism or Asperger Syndrome have challenges that, for most part, remain unrecognised in society. There is one published assessment tool available for girls (Kopp & Gilberg, 2011) containing specific ASSQ-GIRL items and no published assessment tools for adult females. There are currently no research-based interventions for females on the spectrum. There are few professionals worldwide trained with an understanding and experience in working with females on the Autism spectrum. Those of us working in this area know there is currently a deluge of females across the lifespan with undiagnosed Autism struggling with mental health issues and/or co-existing disorders or conditions. It will remain this way for some time into the future.

There is a desperate need all over the world for more trained professionals, more research based on females and comparing females with Autism to their neurotypical peers, more information regarding the internal experiences of a large group of females on the spectrum, more information about the female subtypes, and a huge need for assessment tools, resources, intervention and support designed specifically for females. Current assessment tools do not appear to be suitable or designed to identify particular features of Autism spectrum disorder/condition in females.

It is important to remember that this book is about many adult females who have been misdiagnosed or undiagnosed and as such have not received appropriate or helpful interventions. Poor self-esteem is a common theme, often from early childhood, and the experience of bullying, the later expectations of failing, disapproval by others and/or fear of ridicule.

It is my hope that with earlier diagnoses and interventions, many of the struggles seen in adults today may be avoided, and that appropriate interventions are created to assist females to 'be their own superheroes'.

I Am AspienWoman starts where *I Am AspienGirl*® left, giving voice to the feelings, thoughts, experiences and perceptions of women from a variety of countries, ages and cultures, some diagnosed, some self-diagnosed and many undiagnosed. This book is written for four types of readers. First, for the general population (neurotypical people), to explain the internal experiences and the unique characteristics of adult females with an Autism Spectrum Condition (ASC). Second, this book is written for the female who is just starting her journey to understand that she may too be somewhere on the spectrum herself. Third, for individuals with a formal diagnosis who feel this book may help explain their uniqueness and characteristics to themselves and/or their loved ones through sharing it with family members, partners, friends, colleagues and/or the wider community. Lastly, the book is written for professionals, to assist them in understanding the newly emerging Autistic female phenotype or profile and in their work with their own clients.

I. Use of the word 'Autism' refers to all people on the spectrum including Asperger Syndrome. Autism and Asperger Syndrome are used interchangeably. It also includes those with Pathological Demand Avoidance (PDA) traits.

II. Not all women have the ability to 'mask' their difficulties.

III. Not all women fit the female profile and vice versa. A smaller group of women present with more male characteristics and some males present with more of the female characteristics or presentation.

IV. Whilst all females share the core difficulties and strengths, there exists heterogeneity within the group of females, and as such, many females within the group may be similar to and different from each other. For example, there are females who are introverted and there are females who are extraverted, but all say they struggle socially to some degree. Some females mildly struggle and some females have severe social difficulties.

V. There exists a stereotype of what female Autism is or presents like and it is important to point out that there are many subtypes of females with Autism.

VI. The issue of language and terminology is a contentious one. It is usually the professionals who prefer person first language ("person with Autism") whilst those on the Autism spectrum may prefer "Autistic person". Suffice to say, there is no one way of describing Autism on which everyone can agree on.

The National Autistic Society recently carried out some 'research' on this very topic (a survey) which provided some interesting and contradictory findings. Realising that it is impossible to please everyone on this issue this book prefers to refer to Autism as a condition (Simon Baron Cohen) rather than a disorder (DSM5 terminology). I prefer to use the terms 'Autistic children' and 'Autistic adults', 'Autistic girls' and 'Autistic women and men', 'Autistic women and girls'. I also prefer to use the terms 'women and girls on the Autism spectrum', women on the Autism spectrum', 'girls on the Autism spectrum', 'Autistic adolescents' and /or 'female adolescents on the Autism spectrum'.

As this book goes to print, a groundbreaking study (Nordahl et. al, 2015) is released adding to the growing body of literature suggesting males and females with Autism have different underlying neuroanatomical differences. Research is showing that girls generally display less obvious behavioural symptoms at a young age compared with boys. When compared to typical girls though, girls with Autism have more behavioural and social difficulties. It is my hope that this book may contribute towards 'no more females being left behind'.

Acknowledgements

Thank you to the females and their families, siblings, partners, friends, carers and professionals for sharing their experiences and allowing me to showcase the unique characteristics of Autistic adults, in their own words.

I would like to acknowledge an amazing group of people. They are extraordinary people working in a complex and challenging area and I am most grateful for their support:

Dr Shana Nichols, thank you for your support and providing the foreword to this book. It is an honour and thank you for the valuable work you do for Autistic females.

Dr Temple Grandin, thank you for your support and leading up an inspirational group of remarkable and fascinating Autistic women and thank you for your continued advocacy and strengths-based focus.

Mr Richard Mills, thank you for your support, valuable feedback, your work with the Autism in Pink Project and for your work with and for Autistic females.

I would like to thank each one of the AspienWoman Mentors for agreeing to showcase their talents and act as positive mentors of inspiration for other females on the spectrum:

Dr Temple Grandin, Professor Katherine Milla, Lauren Lovejoy, Jeannette Purkis, Olley Edwards, Jen Saunders, Chou Chou Scantlin, Laura Golden and Deborah Chamberlain, Chelsea Hopkins-Allan, Maja Toudal, Elisabeth Wiklander, April Griffin, Marguerite (Margo) Comeau, Annette Harkness, Megan Barnes, Samantha Craft, Genevieve Kingston, Brandy Nightingale, Shan Ellis Williams, Sybelle Silverpheonix, Dena Gassner, Xolie Morra Cogley, Jessica Ivey and Lexington Sherbin.

I would like to thank the following people for allowing me to showcase their work: Supermodel Samantha Tomlin, Vic of Beachview Photography and Ardent Studios, artist Lexington Sherbin, Annette Stanton Harkness and Bombshell Mandy/Bombshell Pinups and Laney Lane Photography, photographer Christy Maree, April Marie and her gorgeous child and model Kylie and photographer Meg Bitton, Toni Albina for her Alice In Wonderland Mad-Hatter-themed selfie, Dr Temple Grandin and Rosalie Winard, Lauren Lovejoy and photographer Stuart Marsh, Jeanette Purkis and photographer Paul Hagon, Chou Chou Scantlin and photographers Danny Fowler, B.B. Coltrane and Ben P. Powell, Deborah Chamberlain for photos of both Laura Golden and her art, Maja Toudal, photographer Jan Winther and makeup artist Sisse Julin, Elisabeth Wiklander and photographers Benjamin Ealovega and Vanity Studios, London, Marguerite Comeau and photographers Sylvain Boisvert, Garry BJ and Dmitri Moisseev, Megan Barnes and photographer Lann Levinge, Samantha Craft and Wati ProjectLife Photography, Sybelle Silverpheonix and photographers/art by Mike Reilly and Arthur Eisenberg Photography, Xolie Morra and Rusty Cock Ridge Photography, Jessica Ivey and photographers Jarrod Lister and Christopher Sloan.

Thank you to the beautiful Be Your Own Superhero (BYOSH) models: Kayla from Ireland, Ella from Finland, Isabelle from the Netherlands, Chloe from Australia, Jewel from Canada, Kate from Scotland, Johanna from the USA, Shoshanna from Israel, Jennilee Rose from Canada and Anisa from Poland.

Thank you Aniko, Rachel Phillips, Marguerite Comeau and Annette Harkness for the use of your beautiful poems.

I would like to thank the following people for their support and for perusing my drafts and providing me with valuable feedback: Dr Shana Nichols, Dr Temple Grandin, Sarah Hendrickx, Mr Richard Mills, Gareth Morewood, Carol Povey (NAS), Anna Kennedy, Carrie Grant, Rachael Lee Harris, Mari Nosal, Dr Linda Barboa, Dr Jennifer Imig Huffman, Dr Heather MacKenzie, Cynthia D'Agostino, Alison Glover, Lauren Lovejoy and Jo Caspers.

Thank you to the translators who, with their expertise and passion, have made this knowledge and information available to girls and women, their families, supporters and professionals in many other countries.

Thank you to all of you who wrote to me sharing your stories, your struggles and your celebrations.

I would like to acknowledge my professional support team (you know who you are), in addition to Lilly, Lauren Lovejoy, Alison Glover and Natalie Curtis.

Last and certainly not least, I would like to thank Kylee Ellis and her team at the Publishing Queen (www.publishingqueen.com) for their professionalism, support, editing and assistance in this process.

Testimonials

In this sequel to her first book Aspiengirl®, Tania Marshall examines the topic of Autism in women, utilising the personal perspectives of women themselves. Despite a greater awareness of Autism more generally, Autism in girls and women is only just beginning to receive wider attention and the majority remain undetected, in many instances leading unhappy, unfulfilled lives and often struggling to survive. This 'lost generation' of women is only now beginning to have the nature of the condition and needs recognised. Despite the talents and qualities such women may possess, they largely remain disadvantaged and vulnerable. This is often compounded by a lack of self-awareness and awareness by their families and a poorly informed professional community. As with its forerunner the essence of this book is its attractiveness, readability and clarity. It will open the eyes of the reader in so many ways and although adopting a positive tone throughout avoids trivialising or glamourising the topic or pulling its punches, Tania Marshall does not shy away from difficult areas or topics and has sensible approaches to offer. I am sure it will have a wide appeal – from those women who are or suspect they may be on the autism spectrum, families and professionals in many fields such as employment, education, health and social support.

Richard Mills
Research Director, Research Autism, London
Hon. Research Fellow, Dept. Psychology, the University of Bath, UK

There is definitely a need for more information for individuals who get diagnosed later in life. Diagnosis as an adult can provide tremendous insight into why relationships were so difficult. When I was in college, I remember many older, quirky adults who sought me out and helped me. Today many of these people would be diagnosed with either Autism or Asperger's Syndrome. One woman was the associate dean's wife and she gave me many hours of emotional support during difficult social times in college.

Temple Grandin, Author, USA
The Autistic Brain and Thinking in Pictures

I have been fortunate enough to work with a number of young people and their families in the UK and Ireland during the last 20 years. I am also lucky to be involved with practitioner research: previously developing our 'saturation model' for including young people with Autism in mainstream education (Morewood et al, 2011) and most recently considering the impact of interventions through case studies (Bond et al, 2015). This research is vital; however, I always feel I understand most from listening to young people, hearing their stories and talking to their families.

AspienWoman is the latest book from Tania A. Marshall, and a vital addition to the growing knowledge-base about females and Autism. The 'first-hand' accounts throughout the book support the outcomes of our research: a personalised approach is essential. The comprehensive 'real-life' examples support a rapid increase in understanding and allow for a truly unique viewpoint – highlighting strengths and personal characteristics of the women who have contributed, skilfully linked and collated by Tania, drawing on a wealth of personal experience and expertise.

I am reminded of a quote one of our students, Megan, told me once: 'I feel rather positive about my Autism, because it is part of me and without it I would not be me anymore.' Anyone reading AspienWomen will understand immeasurably more after reading it, as I have. I am always learning, from our young people and their families; Tania's contribution to this knowledge will have considerable impact, as I am certain that AspienWoman will for many, many others around the world. Essential reading, if you are directly involved in working with young people, their families or women with Autism, or if you just want to understand more about some of the amazingly talented individuals who have contributed to this amazing work.

Gareth D Morewood
UK Special Educational Needs Coordinator
Honorary Research Fellow, University of Manchester
Associate Editor, Good Autism Practice Journal
www.gdmorewood.com

Tania Marshall has created a groundbreaking book. Most often we hear the voice of the parent or professional; at last we hear the voice of women with Aspergers. AspienWomen can be totally inspiring! Thoroughly recommend.

Carrie Grant
Vocal coach, judge and TV presenter
Judge, BBC 1's Fame Academy and BAFTA award-winning "Glee Club."
Presenter, *The One Show*
Author, bestselling book *You Can Sing*
Mother to two daughters on the spectrum
United Kingdom

Tania, your book is a reflection of the bright and beautiful possibilities that await women on the Autism spectrum. Many had said, "She will grow out of it," but rather, your book shows that "We grow into it," emerging from confusion and misunderstanding into a new appreciation of our unique and powerful profile. *I am AspienWoman* is a celebration in word and picture, affirming our rightful place in the society in which we live!

Rachael Lee Harris
Psychotherapist specialising in women and girls on the Autism spectrum.
Author of *My Autistic Awakening: Unlocking the Potential for a Life Well Lived*

Once again, Tania has provided a visual conversation starter to demonstrate the wide and varied adult presentation of female Autism. Featuring individual profiles of successful Autistic women along with quotes from individuals and family members, this book will help to further increase the understanding that women with Autism are out there – even if they are hard to spot.

Sarah Hendrickx, M.A. (Autism)
Autistic adult
Author of *Women and Girls with ASD, Understanding Life Experiences from Early Childhood to Old Age.* JKP, (2015)

The layout of *I Am AspienWoman* is quite impressive. The photos are vivid. The self-descriptive disclosures regarding living with Asperger's by individuals and family members provide a venue for other women on the spectrum to identify with. The photos and self-disclosures are uniquely reinforced with factual information regarding the bio/psycho/social characteristics of those on the spectrum by the author in a format that the layman can understand. *I Am AspienWoman* takes Asperger's and living on the spectrum out of the clinical context and provides a human and real window into the meaning of living with Asperger's.

I Am AspienWoman focuses on the positive aspects of living with Asperger's. It does not focus on the deficits. For sure, this book portrays the challenges associated with being on the spectrum but the strengths that individuals possess due to having Asperger's is reinforced. This will be resultant in providing hope and the reader perceiving themselves or a family member who has Asperger's in a more positive light.

The unique combination of presenting bios of 'real people', challenges and the strengths of individuals with Asperger's will provide a venue for not only appreciation of strengths but challenges that affect individuals on the spectrum as well. *I Am AspienWoman* cracks the heuristics of society at large and any misnomers regarding Asperger's.

Thank you, Tania, for writing a much needed and 'human' book that many on the spectrum will seek out for positive role models and will cause society at large to change their perception about individuals on the spectrum who they live, love, work and play with on a daily basis.

Mari Nosal M.Ed.
Author
*Ten Commandments Of Interacting With Kids On
The Autism Spectrum And Related Commandments*

When I first read *I am AspienGirl®* last year, I knew immediately that we would be treated to sequels. *I am AspienWoman* takes up where *AspienGirl®* leaves off, taking the concept through a beautiful age progression. AspienWoman does not glamourise Asperger's but rather gives a balanced, factual picture of the strengths and challenges that characterise this population. The short vignettes tell the stories of the lives of real people, told from both the perspective of AspienWomen themselves, and from those who surround them in life. Tania Marshall outlines common traits and needs of the AspienWoman, with which many women will identify.

This book is alive with pictures and stories of beautiful, successful AspienWomen. The focus is on the strength of those spotlighted, and includes personal tips for success from these role models to the reader. Reading the stories of this group of featured role models, it is clear that 'different' does not mean 'less'. Ms Marshall also includes a section of ideas on how a professional might use *I am AspienWoman* to enhance the lives of women with Asperger's.

I am AspienWoman throws a lifeline to young ladies dealing with a feeling of isolation or frustration due to Asperger's Syndrome. Ms Marshall offers a sense of community to this population, along with proof that success and happiness can be a reality for the AspienWoman.

Linda Barboa, PhD
Author of:
Stars in Her Eyes: Navigating the Eyes of Childhood Autism
Tic Toc Autism Clock
Steps to Forming A Disability Ministry
Albert is My Friend series teaching children about autism.

Foreword

Dr Shana Nichols, PhD
**Clinical Psychologist and founder of ASPIRE Center
for Learning and Development in New York, USA
Author of *Girls Growing Up on the Autism Spectrum***

Having written an endorsement for *I Am AspienGirl®*, and recommending it as a must-read to anyone parenting or working with a girl on the Autism spectrum (including the girls themselves), I was delighted to be asked by Tania Marshall to write the foreword for *I Am AspienWoman*.

I began working regularly with AspienGirls in 2005, having developed 'girls only' social coping groups. At that time, there were no resources available for families that specifically addressed the issues faced by females, and limited research had been conducted with the goal of understanding the experiences of girls and women. Few clinicians had begun to specialise in this area, yet those of us who did knew that these girls and women have unique needs and that a subset of females present with behaviours and characteristics that can be quite dissimilar from their male counterparts. When viewed through a 'male' lens, AspienGirls and Women are often overlooked, missed, misdiagnosed and misunderstood, resulting in a rallying call for the professional community to pay attention and work towards remedying the situation.

In recent years that call has begun to be answered. Over 15 studies addressing gender differences and the experiences of females have been published in professional journals in 2015 alone. Attendees at the annual International Meeting for Autism Research in 2015 were able to participate in a session devoted entirely to research concerning females on the Autism spectrum. A number of clinical conferences with the goal of offering practical strategies and facilitating the understanding of females have popped up globally in the last two years, providing the opportunity to learn from professionals and from women on the spectrum themselves. Lastly, the number of books and resources that are available to families, professionals and females has grown. *I Am AspienGirl®* was a rich and unique contribution to this literature, and I am thrilled to say that *I Am AspienWoman* is equally creative and inspiring.

With its characteristic eye-catching photos and powerful quotes from members across the entire female Autism spectrum community, readers of *I Am AspienWoman* will find no shortage of knowledge, illumination and encouragement – after all, an important message of the book is for women to be their own superheroes. *I Am AspienWoman* celebrates the strengths, triumphs, talents and beauty of females, yet does not shy away from a balanced discussion of challenges, concerns, and important yet often overlooked issues such as gender and sexuality, personal safety, mental health and motherhood. Essential themes that run throughout include Identity, Connection, Validation, Self-Care, Inspiration, Strategies and Optimism. Top tips from over 20 Real-life AspienWoman Super-hero Mentors offer a smorgasbord of suggestions and support.

The pages of *I Am AspienWoman* hold a diamond of a message for any reader. It may be big, life changing, and fabulously eye opening. It may touch your heart and whisper "I see you." It may provide the much-needed words to explain, describe or share thoughts, feelings and experiences. It may open doors, or it may give a gentle push to close those that are no longer helpful. It may be a hint of hope, or perhaps a spark of Superhero-ness. It may be all that is needed to get started, re-start or continue on the journey of becoming the best version of who you are: an AspienGirl® or Woman, a family member, a friend, an educator, a professional.

As a field, we still have a long way to go in advocating for better understanding of female Autism, educating and training professionals, developing appropriate assessments and treatments, and creating a community of support and inclusion for AspienGirls and Women. Given all that has happened in the last few years, I am encouraged that we are headed in the right direction. Thankfully there are those special books, like *I Am AspienWoman*, that act as a guide and an incredibly accessible resource. As with her prior book, Tania's latest offering has not surprisingly leaped onto my recommended reading list.

Shana Nichols, PhD
Licensed Clinical Psychologist
Founder and Director
ASPIRE Center for Learning and
Development, New York, USA

Deer

Take my hand and so we run:
We are elk and we are deer,
Lush forest surrounding us,
No big bad wolves dare come near.
For you I'm the summer day,
And my eyes the Sun that burns,
Silver clouds above us fly,
And in our hearts fly the birds.
For yours is a mighty oak:
Towards the sky branches stretch...
But mine is a weathered pine,
In its hollow, Winter nests.
But alas! The full moon cometh,
And I shed my deer disguise,
Wearily climb on the roof,
Lo, hear ye my desperate howls.

Aniko, Hungary

Psychedelic Chameleon

I tried it ... fitting in, you know
I'd change my colour, change my face
From red to blue, from green to pink
Masochistic attempts to belong to some place.

You all thought I was one of you
Whoever 'you' were that day
I'd nod and smile and empathise
'She understands' you'd say.

But then I just knew that enough
Was enough, I couldn't go on anymore
All the colours I'd turned merged into sludge brown
I was lost and fatigued to the core.

I thought about fading away into nothing
But then I began to see
All the times that I'd changed to try to match them
All those colours belong to me

And now when I stand, being me, being proud
Whole rainbows of colours appear
I belong to myself, I fit in where I want
Psychedelic Chameleon, I'm here!

Rachel Phillips, United Kingdom

Who am I?

As early as I can remember, I have felt different … from another planet, time or era.
I can remember feeling different and somehow separate from very early on, an observer of others at times.

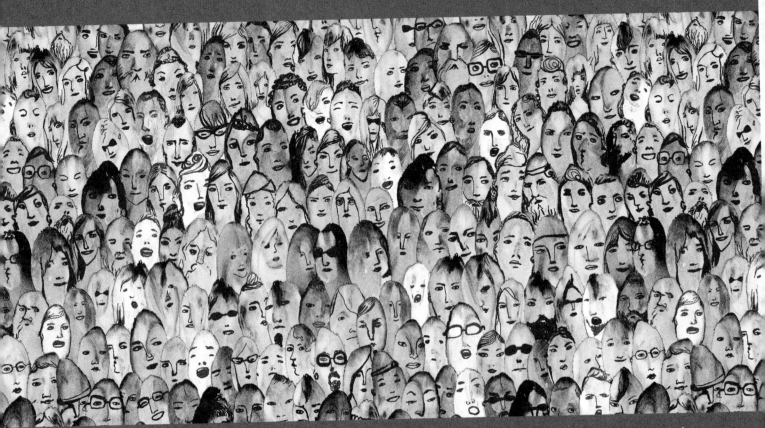

From early childhood, there were a myriad of ways that her differences and oddities were apparent, to me. Yet everyone said I worried too much and she would grow out of it.

– Mother of 25-year-old, recently diagnosed

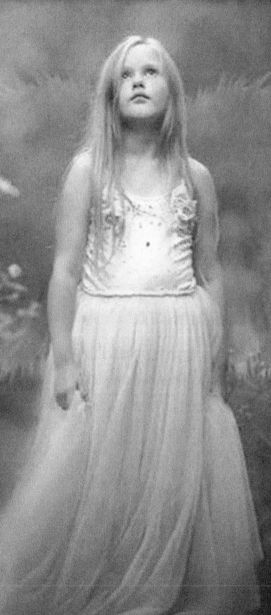

I think all of the time. The thinking just never stops. When I was younger I asked my mum if there was an 'off' button and she said she didn't know what I was talking about!

There has always been something quite angelic and different about her from birth. She is unique, quirky, caring, thinks way too much and loves nature and animals; and the thinking and the questions, they are endless. We call her the 'thinker'.

– Grandparents of 19-year-old teen philosopher

Model: Kylie
Photographer: Meg Bitton

As a group of females, we can be found in a variety of countries, age groups, colours and races. Even though there are millions of us, the feeling of being 'alone' is common. Many of us are from the 'lost generation' and are just discovering why we are so good at some things and not so good at others. Our brains are wired differently.

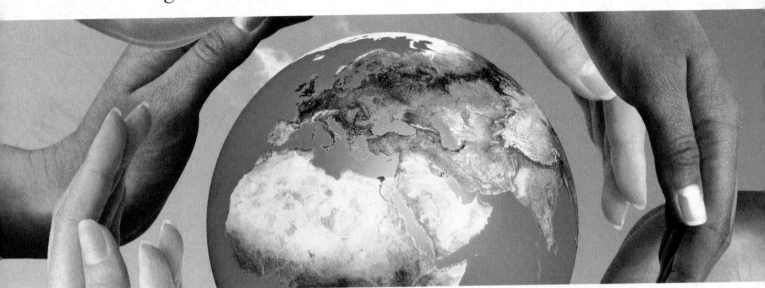

The 'lost generation' is the generation generally born before 1980, the very late diagnosed adults. There is very little known about adult female Autism or Asperger Syndrome. There is approximately 1 in 100 adults with Autism, most of them undiagnosed. They were left behind and often struggled through school silently, dropped out or spent time in mental health facilities.

– Autism psychologist

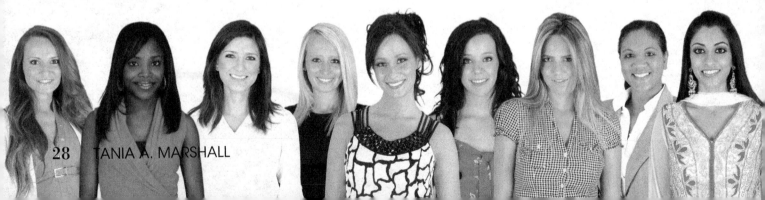

I have recently discovered I have adult female Asperger Syndrome, a form of Autism, a neurological condition from birth. It means I have a 'spikey profile'. I am really good at some things and not so good at others things. I am 46 years old now and just realised that Autism is the explanation for why I am unique, have many strengths and some challenges. Unfortunately, my family still just think I'm 'mad', 'eccentric', 'a weirdo', oh and much worse. I now view myself as 'neurodivergent' rather than a 'freak'. That's a much nicer label for me. I am an AspienWoman. I see, experience and think about the world differently.

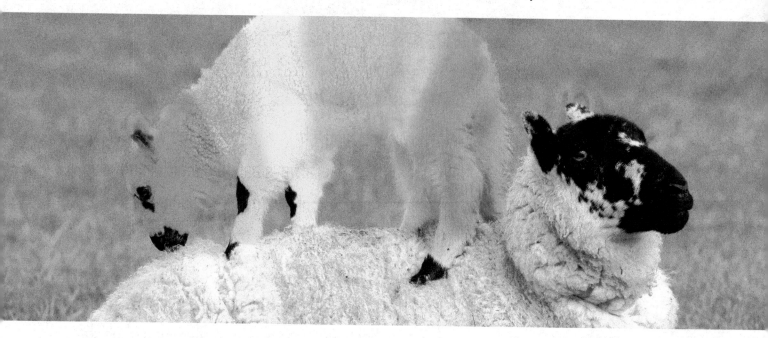

Asperger Syndrome is a newly recognised condition and even newer in females. We have learnt that there are many more adult females on the Autism spectrum than previously thought and that the gender statistics are closer to 2:1. The heterogeneity and subtypes seen in the female presentation makes it quite a complex condition. The DSM5 does acknowledge that girls without intellectual impairment or language delay may go unrecognised, perhaps because of subtler manifestation of social and communication difficulties (page 57).

– Psychologist and researcher

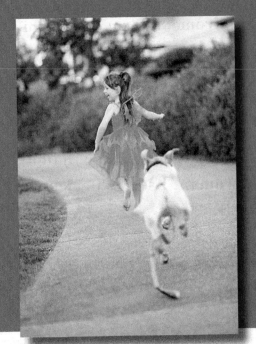

I have always been a bit of a loner and regarded as 'different' or 'reserved' and introverted by others. I often feel like I can never quite fully connect socially with others and I love my animals. Some of my early memories consisted of having trouble with other people's emotions and my own, feeling very anxious, loving the feeling of my stuffed bear. Back then I was sent to a psychologist who said I was "just shy" and I just needed to come "out of my shell".

Christy Maree Photography

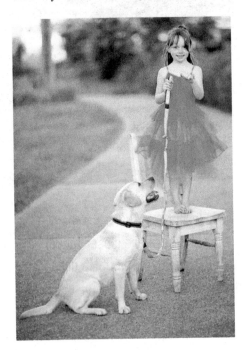

When she was young, she spent more time with the dog than with us. She was always acting out different roles as she grew up. She took drama all throughout school. She has been a professional actress for many years and is really good at it. She has won a variety of acting awards. Her outside image (the one she portrays to the world and in her movie roles) is a combination of all she has observed from other females and other actors in her life. Growing up she was the type to stand on the chair rather than sit on it!

– Mother of 35-year-old professional actress and performer

I cannot remember a time when I wasn't daydreaming, coming up with ideas and being goal-oriented and living in my head. I would imagine I was a certain actor or actress and practise scenes from movies. I would say I am independent, a bit of a rebel … ok … I'll admit it, I've been known to be a rebel and I am described by my mother as a 'nonconformist'.

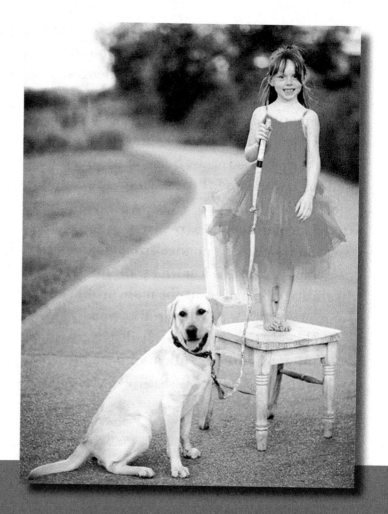

She often goes against the grain and expectations, is strong-willed and nonconformist, sometimes digging her heels in and resisting going along with the crowd. Now that I think back on it, yup, one of our struggles was that she was so nonconformist. Now this is the quality that has made her such an excellent actress.
– Mother of professional actress, model and animal whisperer

What makes us as a group so complex is that we can be quite different from each other, yet have similar talents and challenges. Some of us experience mild sensory, social or communication issues and function well and some of us experience some of these characteristics severely. Some of us function well for a while and then we cannot function at all for a few weeks. Autism also tends to be a condition of extremes. For many of us, you would have no idea from looking at us. That is why it is known as an 'invisible' disability. Some of us fit the male profile and some males fit the female profile. Some of us also have other conditions or disorders in addition to Autism. Talk about complex!

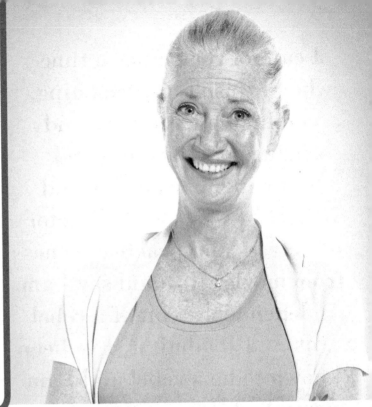

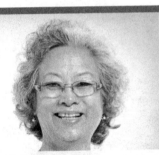
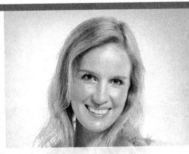
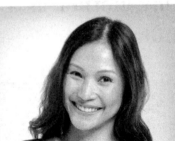
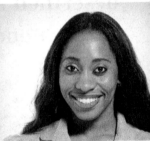

I have met many females of all ages and a variety of cultures. Some of them are formally diagnosed, some have an inkling about why they are different, many have been misdiagnosed, many are self-diagnosed with no way of obtaining a formal diagnosis, and many females have lived and died not knowing their brains were wired differently.

– Tania A. Marshall, psychologist

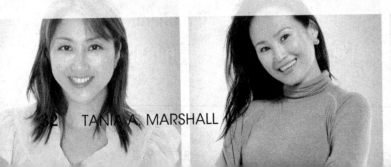
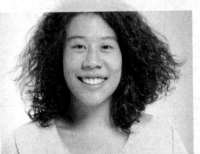
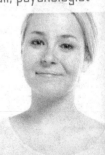

As a family, we have recently discovered that Asperger Syndrome runs in our family. We went to see a specialist for our youngest one, who received a formal diagnosis of Asperger Syndrome, to help her in school. We would have never imagined leaving the clinic with the knowledge that all three of us are on the spectrum! That has answered many questions for us and we are now beginning to feel closer as a family.

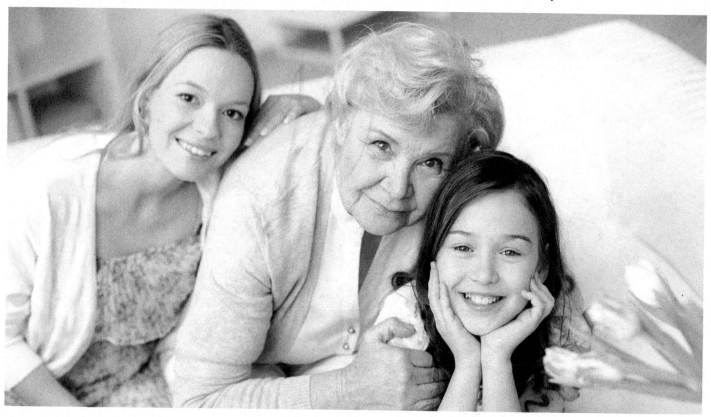

Asperger Syndrome and Autism are neurodevelopmental conditions in which many females have superior attention to detail, a superior memory, the ability to be hyperfocused in a narrow area of interest, and/ or maybe talented at dates and numbers or be gifted in artistic, scientific or technical areas. They may be verbal, visual or pattern thinkers or a combination. Autism tends to make this group of females incredibly good at some things and not so great at other things. They are not better or worse than anyone else, just different ... neurodiverse or neurodivergent.

– Autism researcher

I AM Aspien Woman®   33

I learned there is more than one type of Autism and that there is not a single cause. Both genetic and/or environmental factors play a role and we have no control over them. My psychologist recently told me it is not my fault or my parents, my grandparents or my great-grandparents. I told her I have had a long-term feeling of being constrained by the box. I couldn't – no, I can't – function in the box. It stifles my creativity, my soul, my ability to function … my everything.

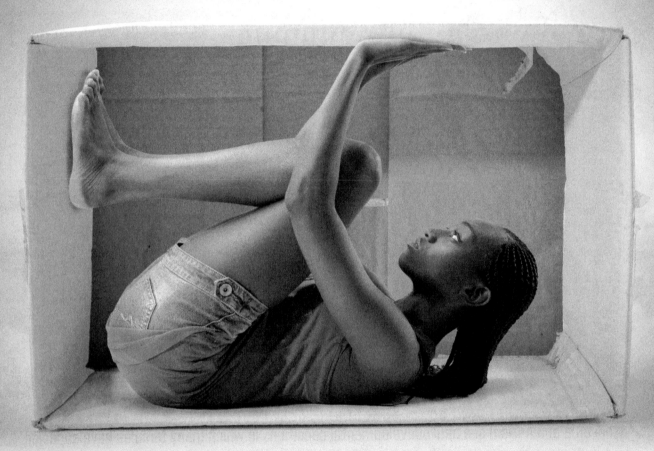

It is common for me to be referred females who do not appear to categorically fit any diagnostic box or criteria. They often do not fit the 'male criteria' of Asperger's and many do not receive the appropriate diagnosis. The current diagnostic criteria, assessment tools and much of the research has a strong 'male-bias'. Many of them have no professionals who understand female Autism, no place, no home, no box, no understanding and no supports.

We really are just starting to learn about female Autism and who this group of talented females are, who tend to have enormous struggles and huge potential, given the right environmental fit.

– Tania A. Marshall, psychologist

Sometimes I wonder how I am still here. Life has always seemed so much harder for me than it is for other people. My peers just glide on by and here I am still trying to grow up. One of my best friends just got engaged and I'm still not interested in boys. I'm always one or two steps behind. My friends all had cars before me. I have a car but I still have to get my licence. Now they are married. I'm still in university. They got their degrees years ago. How did I fall so behind everyone?

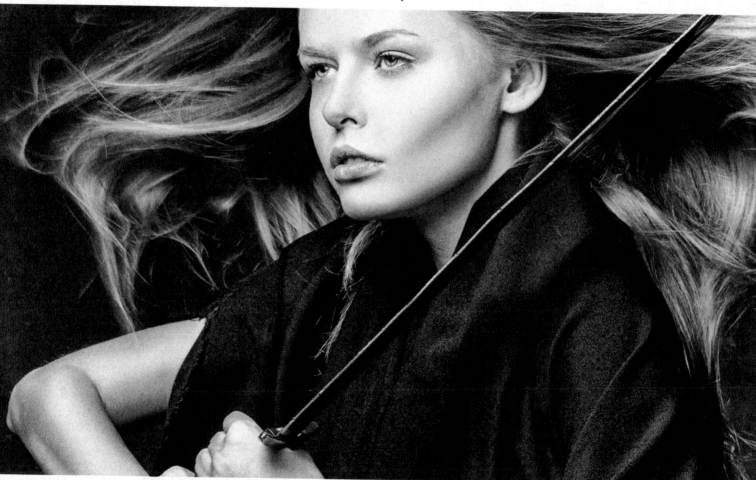

To us, she is a 'Warrior'. She has been through depression, panic attacks, suicidal thoughts, an eating disorder and many failed social relationships. Even the professionals are amazed she is still here. I remember her as a toddler. Back then, we didn't admire her determination and stubbornness so much. That part was a constant battle as parents, but you should see her now. We can see how her strong will is helping her with her life.

– Mother of successful 35-year-old philosophy doctoral candidate

I am an Autistic adult and my Autism is a part of who I am. As a child I had imagined I would grow up and at some magical age be like everyone else. I spent some time in hospitals and have now finally realised that I'm not going to grow out of it.

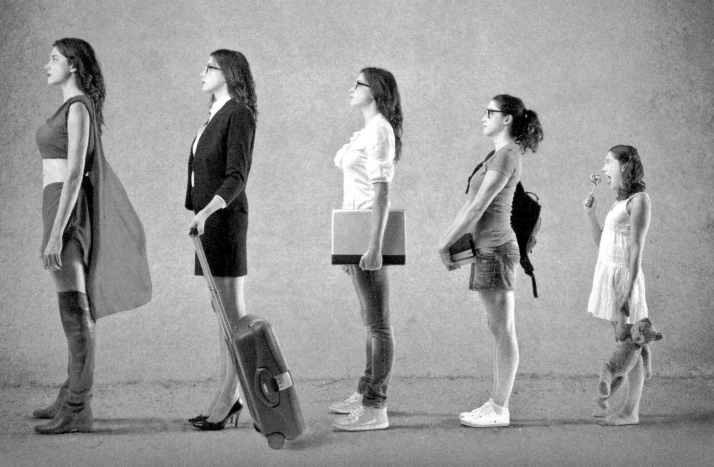

She has always been different, special ... born this way. We recently received the book *I Am AspienGirl®* and it described her to a T, as a young girl. We all knew she was different and now we know **why**. It is the **why** that has helped our family to heal. She is a female with Asperger Syndrome. Most importantly, *she* knows why. We think she is a superhero.

— Mother of recently diagnosed young adult with Autism

Cognitive Style/ Personality Type

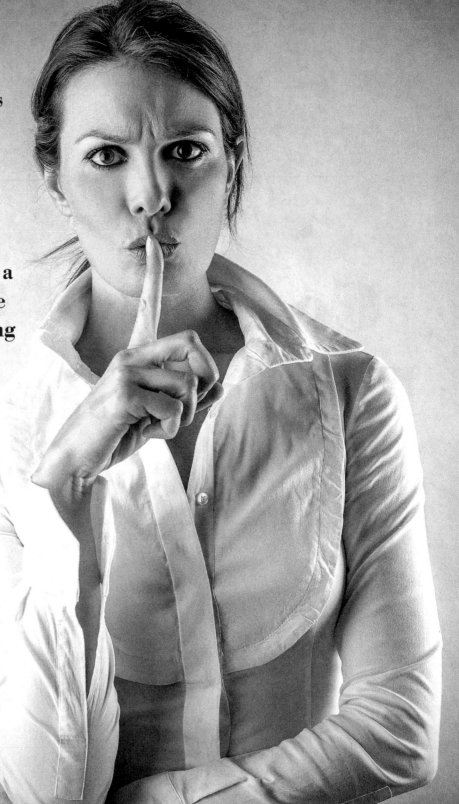

I love the quiet. I need solitude and peace. This type of environment is what I need to survive. I used to live in the concrete jungle, then I moved out into nature and I can't tell you what a difference this has made to me. I do not miss living in the city at all.

> She loves solitude. She is an introvert muse and a highly successful published author. She's very quirky and she often says to us that she needs solitude and quiet so she can hear what the characters of her books are saying to her. Apparently, we're always interrupting her!
> – Mother of writer and best-selling author

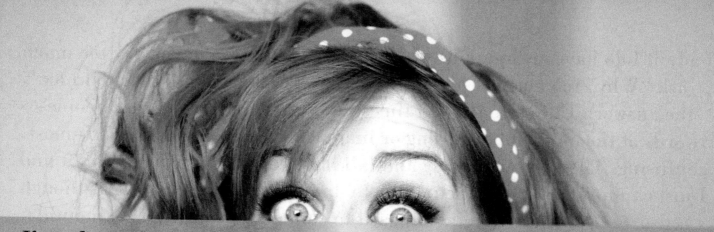

I've always liked things that are unique, different or quirky. I get bored easily with the mundane things in life. I like other people who are like me and want more friends. They are interesting, unique, different, creative … once I can get past my crippling social anxiety and negative self-talk.

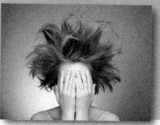

She's a bit of a contradiction really. She's this shy, fashionable and gorgeous young woman, but her style draws so much attention to herself. People have always been drawn to her socially because of her quirkiness, her looks, or superficial sociability. She can be pretty good at small talk too. She has had years of practice. She loves fashion and people want to be around her all the time. She says she can't cope with all the attention.

– Aunt of quirky fashion designer and anxious female overcoming her fears

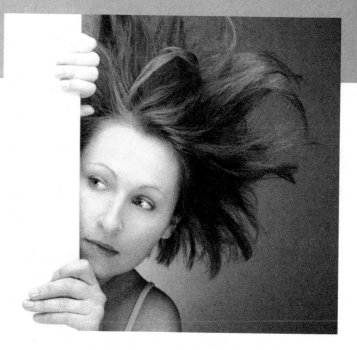

I admit I do have my opinions. At times, I can talk too much, say too much, ask "Why" too much (I just want to know "Why?" and I need to know the answer). Unfortunately, at times my words crash into other people's words at the most embarrassing or inappropriate moments, and it's most confusing. Then I keep talking and talking and talking trying to fix it and I just cannot stop. I have frequently told my parents that it feels as though a neuron is missing that is supposed to connect my brain to my mouth!

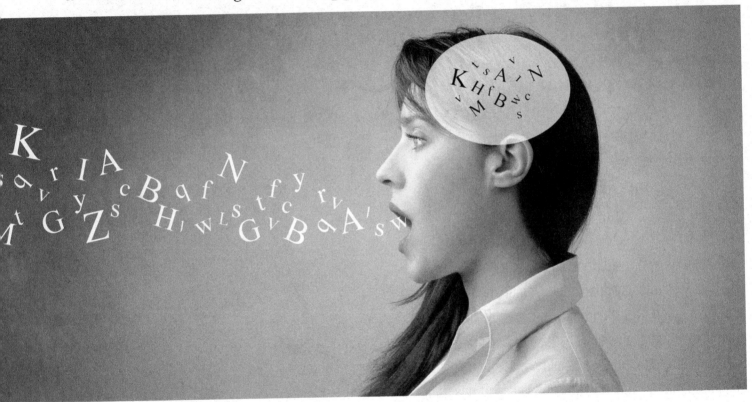

I'm not sure my twin sister realises this (she says she does) but her strong opinions are off-putting to a lot of people. She has some interesting ideas about how people should act and how the world should be, how people should be treated, how she should be treated by others and she tells them! I mean, growing up I remember her following me to the bathroom and sitting outside the bathroom door arguing her point with me!
— Twin sister of AspienWoman with strong opinions

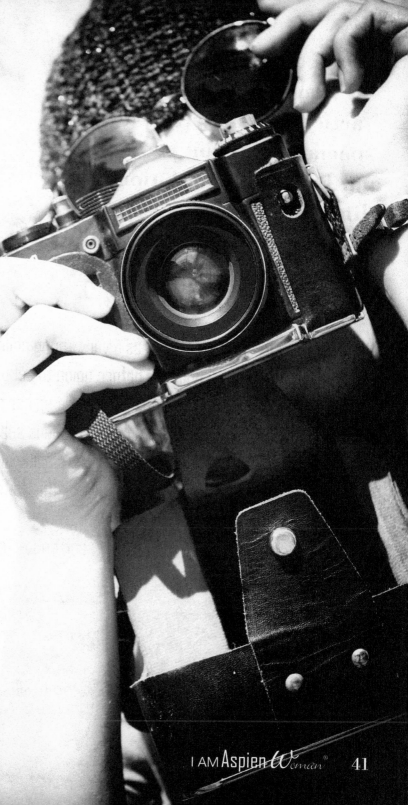

There are positives and negatives to having Autism. Being artistic and creative are parts of my Autism that I really like. Thinking in pictures helps me create and thinking in words is not my strong point. My thoughts are more like visual images and emotions. I think or remember things by going through my mental imagery files, just like computer files, and when I find the folder, it's in moving images and feelings.

She used to always use this word, the 'watcher', saying she felt that she was seeing and looking at others but that it was near impossible for her to be 'with' or 'inside' the group. Now, after all these years, as a professional photographer who loves her job, she is still the 'watcher'. She is a visual thinker who struggles with theoretical and conceptual ideas.

— Father 'of AspienWoman
self-employed photographer

I am a word-fact thinker.
I am a highly verbal,
articulate university-level
special-education professor
and I also do translation and
linguistics work as I speak
three languages. I am really
good at those things and not
so great at drawing.

We knew she was special because as a very young child she started speaking other languages before going to school. She can recall all kinds of facts and even made up her own fairy language with a symbol for each letter. She is self-taught and learns them just like osmosis; she's a learning junkie. She is a professor and a translator for the United Nations now and loves her work.

– Impressed father of university professor and translator

I am a musician, composer and forensic accountant. I love numbers and mathematics. I am a pattern thinker. My work involves lots of spreadsheets, and I'm able to see patterns and solve problems other people can't see so clearly. I'm now a forensic accountant. They love me because I find them money. I love it because I get to figure things out. I've been called a walking computer, oh and a great detective. I'm also good at music and math.

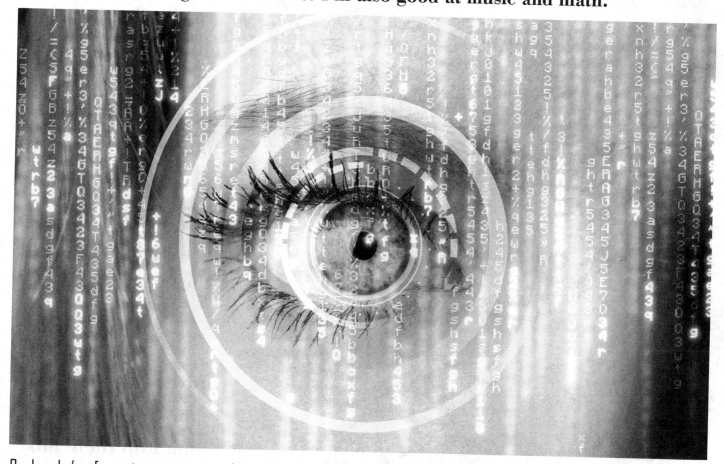

By day she's a forensic accountant and at night she plays in the Philharmonic orchestra. She does find social interactions exhausting but thankfully both her careers allow her enough solitude that she doesn't burn out. Playing music is soothing for her. Her psychologist taught her, and us, all about 'extreme self-care' and why it's so important for all of us.

– Mother of talented accountant, musician and self-professed workaholic

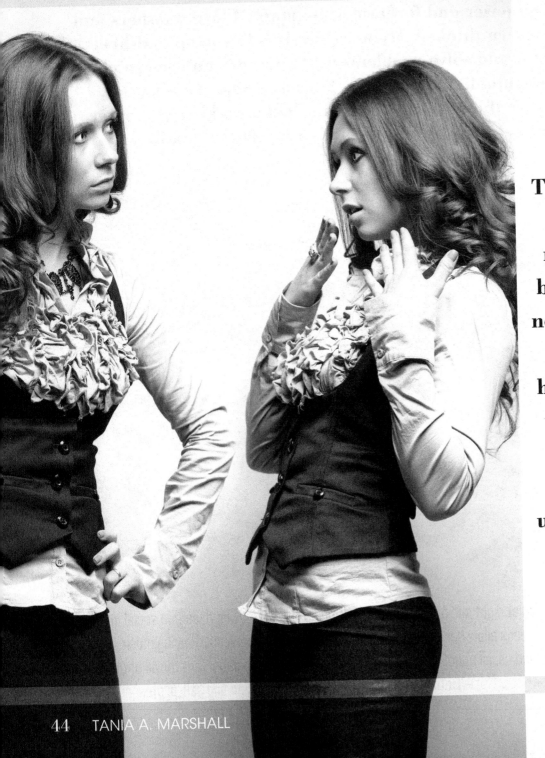

I'm still trying to understand why people see me as a 'perfectionist'. They say I have high expectations for myself and others, but I think they just need to work harder. They are even hinting that I attend the 'perfectionism' group therapy sessions at my university. Me? Well, most people just don't do their job right!

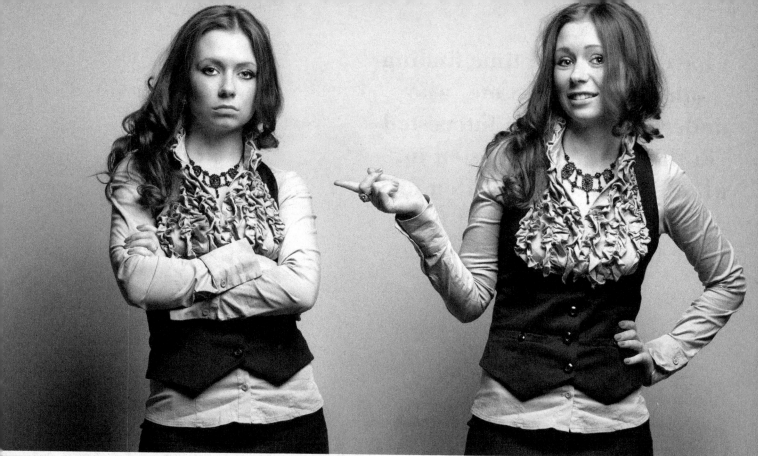

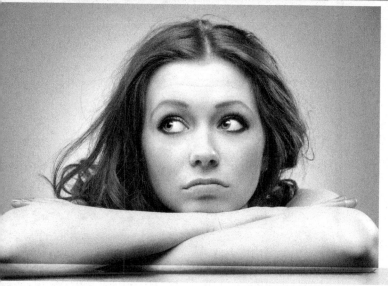

She has always been very hard on herself. She is the first to give herself a time-out. When she was younger she even told on herself to her teachers. She doesn't take criticism or feedback well, but the irony is she loves to dish it out to others. She has gotten into trouble for being a 'tattle-tale', is often plagued by negative thinking, often too serious at times, is described as 'intense' in everything she does and is prone to burning out and 'disappearing' for a while. We joke about her 'disappearing tricks' and her 'invisibility cloak', but since her diagnosis we now understand her.

– Parents of newly diagnosed young adult

I have had a hard time finding other people like me, who understand me, are interested in things I am interested in, who think like me. I often feel like there is no one out there like me and I can feel alone even in a crowd.

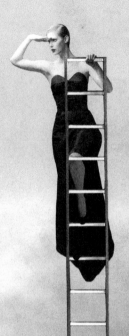

Her expectations are very high. Not many people can keep up to her level of tenacity and commitment to her goals or the rules. She is often frustrated with others for not 'measuring up' to her self-imposed rules. She has achieved every goal she has set her mind on and is one of the best doctoral students I have ever supervised.

– Professor of Engineering and doctoral supervisor

I have a high sense of justice. This used to get me in a lot of trouble as a child and teenager, in the classroom and at home. It still does at times, even now, as an adult. I just love debating and arguing. Sometimes I find myself arguing when there is no point or just for the sake of it. It just comes out of my mouth and has got me in trouble on more than one occasion!

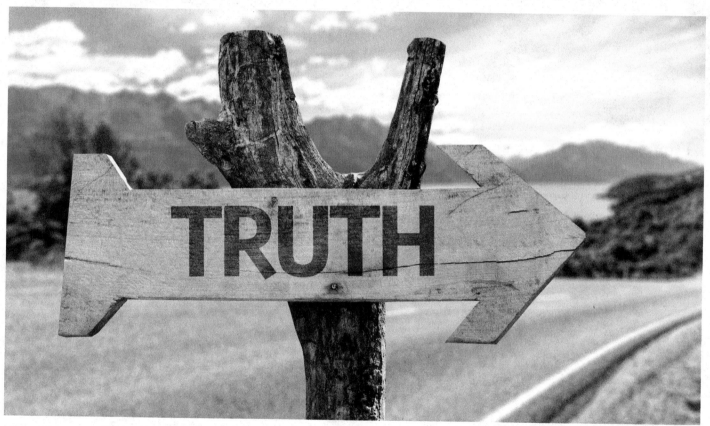

We have always said somewhere in her brain is an enlarged justice gland! She has a strong moral and ethical code and loves to debate. When she was younger she took it too far and got into trouble with the law. She would get herself in trouble because she did not understand that other people's business is not her business and she needed to stay out of it. Her sense of superiority over others was not one of her best features in her teens. Now, as a lawyer, she can channel her 'inner DIVA' in court where she is more successful.

– Father (and lawyer) of AspienWoman lawyer and truth seeker

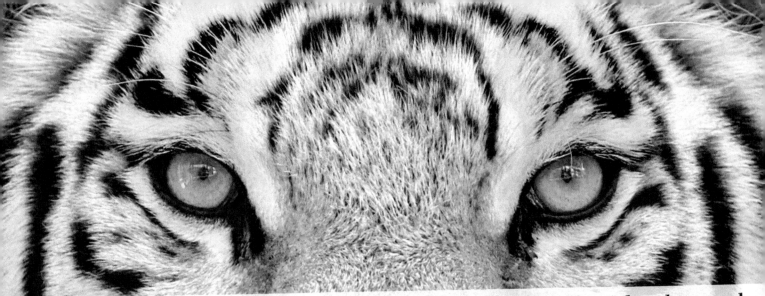

I am an animal analyser, an animal behaviourist and have always loved to watch animals (since I was a little girl) and imagine what they were thinking about and why they were doing what they were doing. And now I do it for a living as a zoologist (and teach about it as a college professor)! I love working at the zoo. They're my kind. I don't work so well with other people.

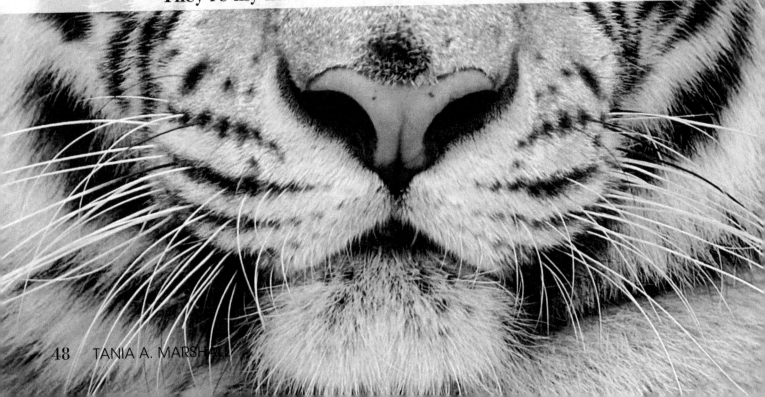

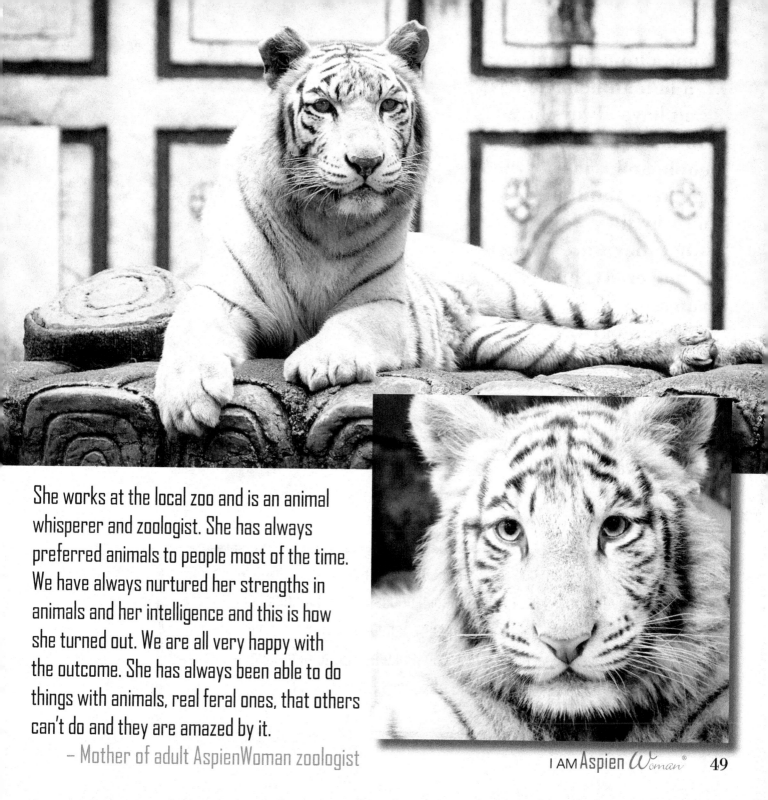

She works at the local zoo and is an animal whisperer and zoologist. She has always preferred animals to people most of the time. We have always nurtured her strengths in animals and her intelligence and this is how she turned out. We are all very happy with the outcome. She has always been able to do things with animals, real feral ones, that others can't do and they are amazed by it.

– Mother of adult AspienWoman zoologist

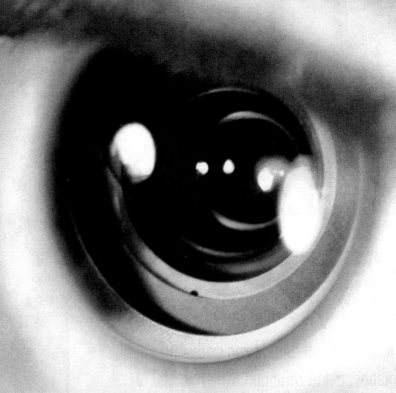

I am a human analyser
... a human behaviourist
and have always loved
to observe and watch
people and imagine what
they were thinking about
and why they were doing
what they were doing.
In university, one of my
professors was a forensic
psychologist. I took
psychology in university
and now I do it for a living.
I worked in the police
force for a while and now I
work in counter-terrorism.

Females on the spectrum can be found in many helping professions including psychiatry, psychology, social work, special education, the medical profession, nursing and/or teaching. Some women with Asperger Syndrome, *with a particular profile of characteristics*, can make exceptional federal or undercover agents, profilers, or parts of special force teams.

– Autism psychologist

Subtypes

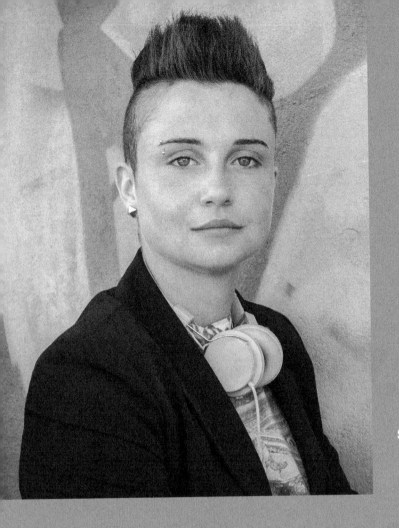

From my earliest memories, I considered myself a tomboy and wore t-shirts and jeans all the time. loved my jeans, shirts and climbing trees (although getting down was anything but glamorous). My mum hated the way I dressed and I just did not get how to be; I mean, how do you 'BE' a girl? I didn't get the whole makeup thing, doing hair and being 'girly' girl. I often wondered, "How come I don't know all this?" I cannot wear socks, love my hair short, cannot wear wool or scratchy clothes, and I cut out all clothing labels.

She couldn't care less about fitting in at all. She never has and I don't think she ever will. She is a tomboy extravert and was born to stand out. She hates a lot of things about this world. She thought the girls in school were stupid, talked about nothing; holding hands and gossiping was pointless. They hated her because she was different. Males are much easier to get along with, for her. In terms of her peers, she has always been an outcast and this has really affected her self-esteem.

Mother of 19-year-old tomboy

I did make friends with some of the neighbourhood kids. I was an oddball who didn't fit in, who loved animals, reading, music and art with a passion. Every Christmas I am still reminded of how upset I got with the kids for killing bugs and apparently I fought very hard for the rights of the firefly, insects and bugs to live a life free of fear from humans. I'd think, "How do you 'BE' a kid? I've never felt like a kid". I loved being with the adults. Now, I have no idea how to 'BE' an adult.

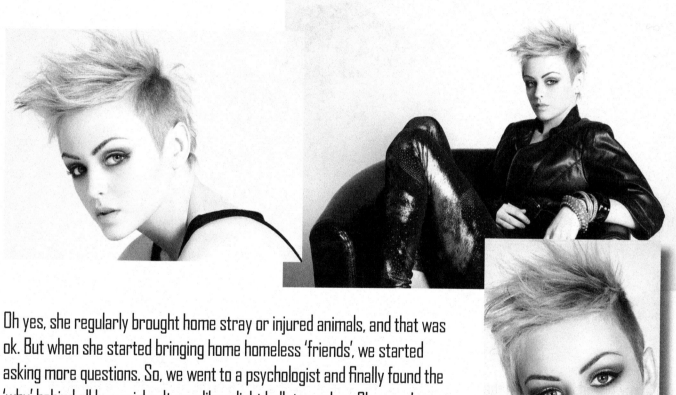

Oh yes, she regularly brought home stray or injured animals, and that was ok. But when she started bringing home homeless 'friends', we started asking more questions. So, we went to a psychologist and finally found the 'why' behind all her quirks. It was like a light bulb turned on. She now has a diagnosis of Autism, is in university and now volunteers at the local zoo. She still lives in her own world and literally believes she's a fairy rather than a human but thankfully has now stopped telling people that!

– Parents of unconventional, quirky animal-loving university student

I am a private kind of person, the quiet one; I was, no ... I still am painfully shy, highly sensitive, introverted, and those were the first 'labels', then that changed to social anxiety, depression and an eating disorder. From a very young age I was a very passive personality and self-conscious, trying my best to be liked or go unnoticed. I tried very hard to blend into the walls whenever I could. I don't like attention.

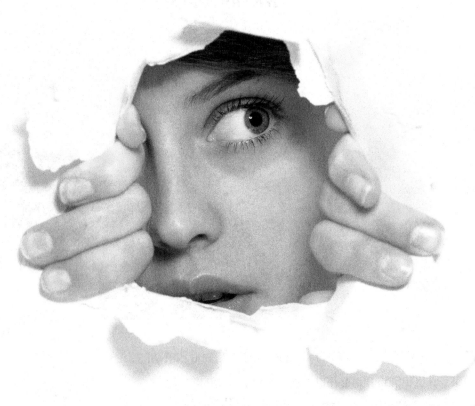

I describe my granddaughter as the Queen of Understatement with a delicate disposition. Most of the time she says nothing ... she just has nothing to say. If she says something you know it's important. We've always wondered what goes on in that marvellous brain of hers. She is a successful artist, who is still learning to manage her anxiety. She speaks more through her art and is quite difficult to get to know.

– Grandfather of guarded and private Aspienwoman

I really identify with being a bookworm. I love reading, learning and books. I mean, I have 1000 books, all catalogued, already in my specially made library my dad made me. Books are my friends. I live in sweat pants and workout gear or t-shirt and jeans. I dress more for comfort than for fashion. I dress up if I have to go out but I can't wait to come home and take off the makeup, heels and scratchy clothing.

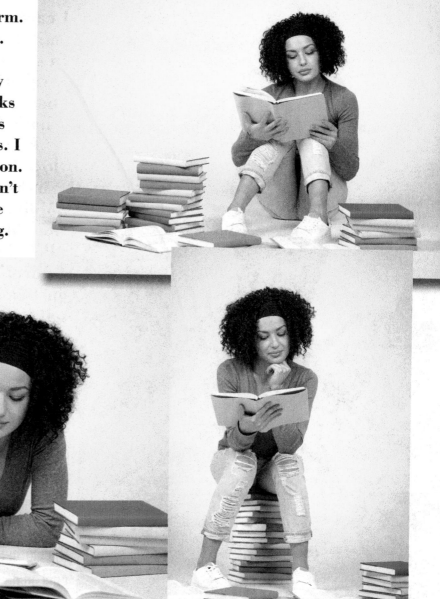

She is a bookworm and a professional student, always learning. I swear she was born with a book in her little baby hands. She has a master's degree in library studies and I am really proud of her.

– Mother of librarian daughter

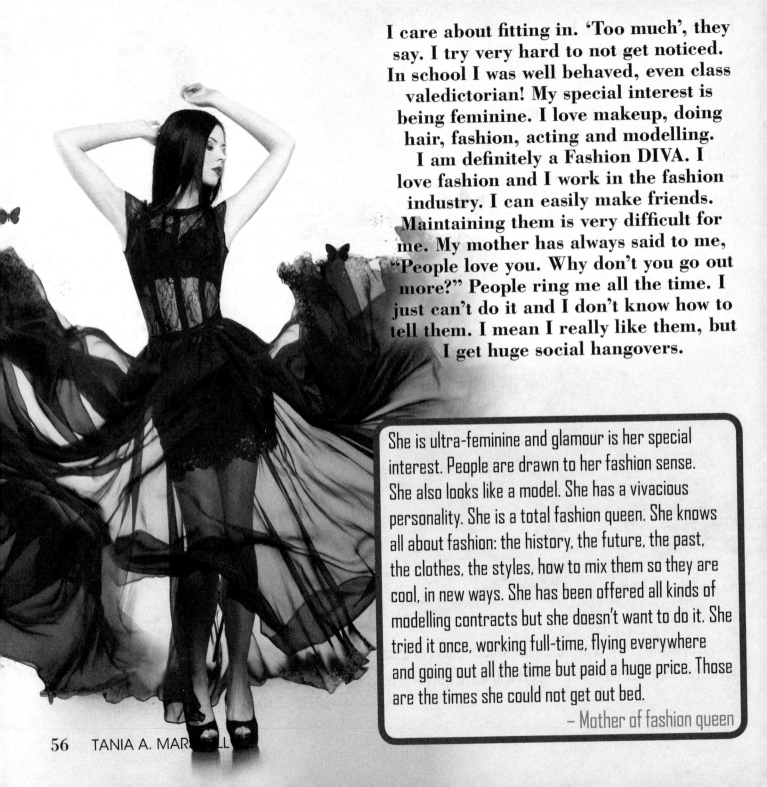

I care about fitting in. 'Too much', they say. I try very hard to not get noticed. In school I was well behaved, even class valedictorian! My special interest is being feminine. I love makeup, doing hair, fashion, acting and modelling.

I am definitely a Fashion DIVA. I love fashion and I work in the fashion industry. I can easily make friends. Maintaining them is very difficult for me. My mother has always said to me, "People love you. Why don't you go out more?" People ring me all the time. I just can't do it and I don't know how to tell them. I mean I really like them, but I get huge social hangovers.

She is ultra-feminine and glamour is her special interest. People are drawn to her fashion sense. She also looks like a model. She has a vivacious personality. She is a total fashion queen. She knows all about fashion: the history, the future, the past, the clothes, the styles, how to mix them so they are cool, in new ways. She has been offered all kinds of modelling contracts but she doesn't want to do it. She tried it once, working full-time, flying everywhere and going out all the time but paid a huge price. Those are the times she could not get out bed.

– Mother of fashion queen

I would describe myself as an academic and research superstar. I love learning and I am an extravert who loves to talk, too much at times, or so they tell me. I also love to debate. I have been attached to a university for years now. I don't ever want to leave, except to time travel back to live in the Jane Austen era. I absolutely adore English literature, Shakespeare, anything Victorian. I have always loved words, grammar, *Pride and Prejudice* …

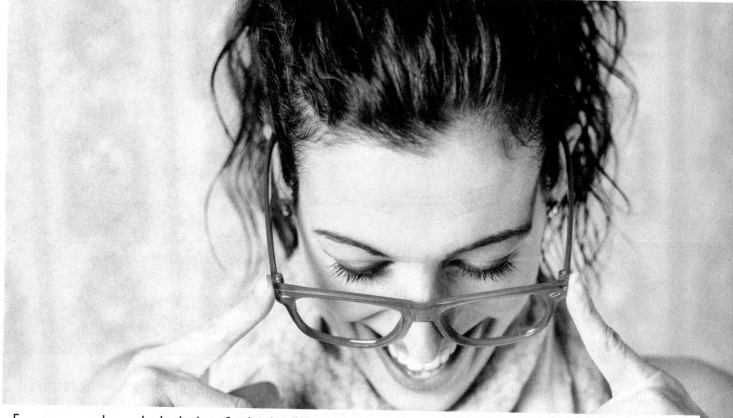

From very early on she had a love for books. She could read before she went to school, didn't like sharing her books or people touching or opening them. She would rather stay at home and read a good book than go out.

– Grandparents of literature expert

I am an ultra-competitive athlete ... even with myself. It is WHO I am. People ask me what am I training for? I tell them 'life'. I run two to three hours a day plus weights and counting calories is really important to me. I need to train. When I don't train I'm very anxious. I love my routine.

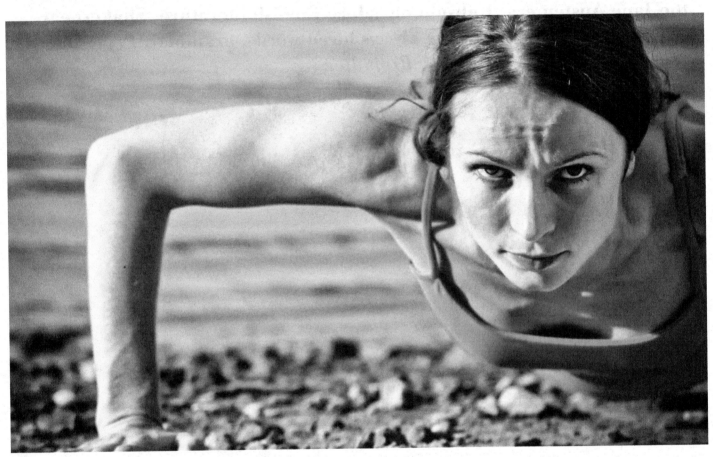

She was made for this ... this something ... if we knew what it was. I mean, she is highly competitive, determined, focused on her goals and everything revolves around her sport and training. She is quite addicted to working out. We asked her recently what she was training for and she said, "Oh I'm not competing for anything!" If she can't get in her workout she gets very stressed. We think she uses exercise as a habit to control her life and it's a ritualistic daily, often twice daily, event for her.   – Parent of 24-year-old in training and competing for life

I am a domestic **DIVA**. I love cooking, organising dinners and get-togethers at my place. I love having people around, just not so much interacting with them, so I stay busy arranging, rearranging, sorting, helping, making sure everyone is watered and fed. Fussing over everyone is what I love to do.

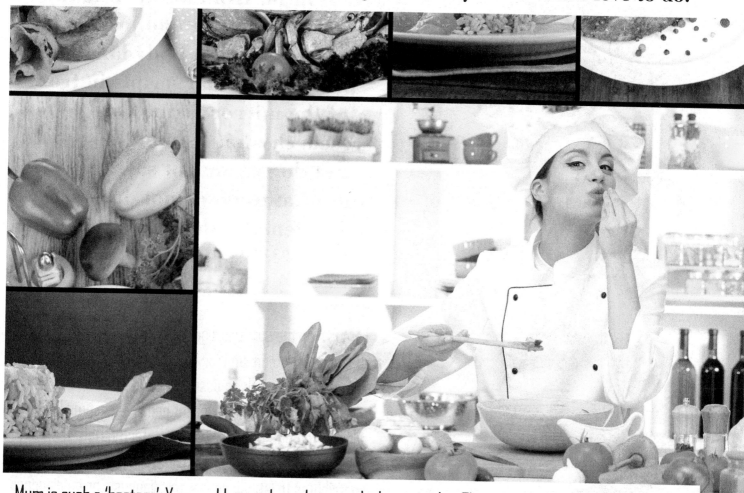

Mum is such a 'hostess'. You would never know how much she struggles. There are times where she just cannot leave the house. She has the groceries delivered, other supplies, everything delivered. We think she might have agoraphobia because she seldom leaves the house and has a lot of anxiety.

– Daughter of amazing cook, mother and housewife

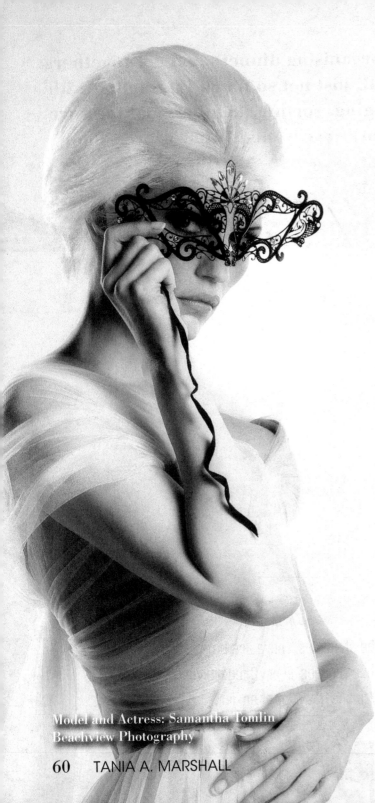

I am the consummate chameleon and blender. I have used all kinds of strategies over the years to fit in: from mimicking my peers, studying and practising social skills and body language, practising social scripts in front of the mirror, using Google to research what I should or should not do, say or not say. I figure out what to do or not do, observe other females then copy or mimic them.

Females on the spectrum generally lack a strong sense of self, self-esteem and/or identity. Their ability to use chameleon-like skills to assimilate and be involved with a variety of groups or different people over time has allowed them to fit in, for a time. Unfortunately, the mask often falls off and it can be this very strategy that contributes to late diagnosis, misdiagnosis or no diagnosis at all. The 'chameleon' type is one of the least likely to receive a diagnosis due to the ability to blend into any environment. This is also the type most likely to receive invalidation from others after their diagnosis.

– Tania A. Marshall, psychologist

Model and Actress: Samantha Tomlin
Beachview Photography

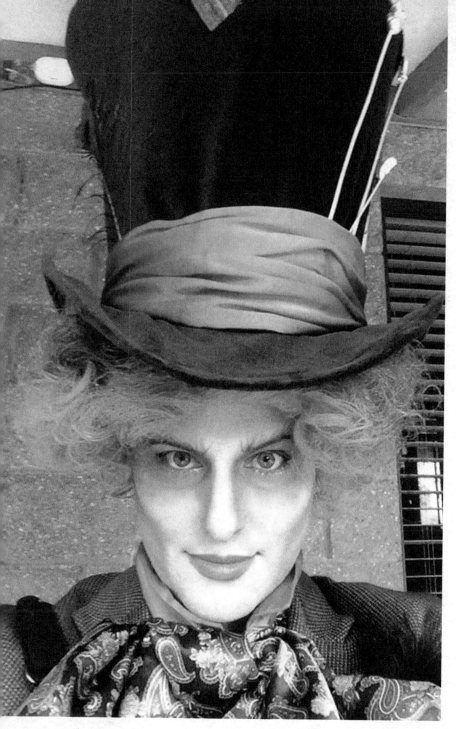

Toni Albina, Selfie
Inspired by The Mad Hatter

Studying drama and being an actor brought a real comfort and solace because I have never really had any idea who I am. I can dive straight into a new world or become a new character which people would love. I do feel concerned at times that I have never had a solid concept of my identity. I do live mainly in fantasy and I would prefer to live in a different time, planet or era. When I was a child, it was okay to be a fairy princess. Unfortunately, I'm now an adult and that's not an easy career option to get into!

From very early on she has been an actor. She was singing before she could speak and pretending to be animals and fairies when she was a toddler!

– Mother of actor in musical theatre

For as long as I can remember, I have been on a quest for self-understanding and self-improvement. I am driven to figure myself and other people out. I have analysed myself as far back as I can remember, reanalysed myself, been to many psychologists, psychiatrists, doctors and psychics. I love self-help books, courses, anything to improve myself. My special interest is self-improvement, quantum physics, medicine, anything to do with bettering oneself and self-help.

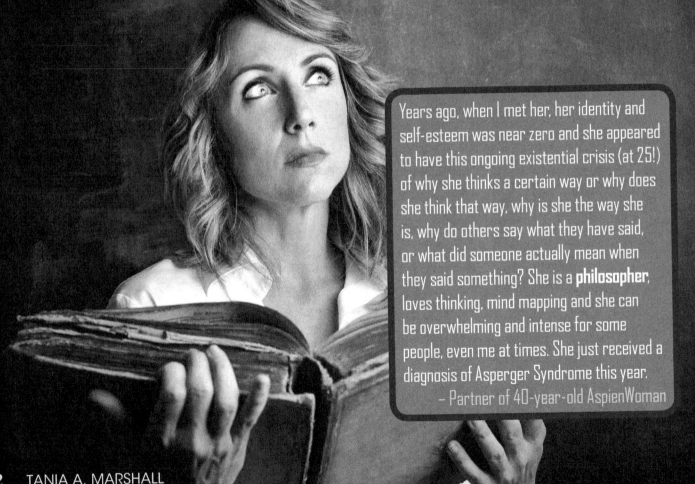

Years ago, when I met her, her identity and self-esteem was near zero and she appeared to have this ongoing existential crisis (at 25!) of why she thinks a certain way or why does she think that way, why is she the way she is, why do others say what they have said, or what did someone actually mean when they said something? She is a **philosopher**, loves thinking, mind mapping and she can be overwhelming and intense for some people, even me at times. She just received a diagnosis of Asperger Syndrome this year.

– Partner of 40-year-old AspienWoman

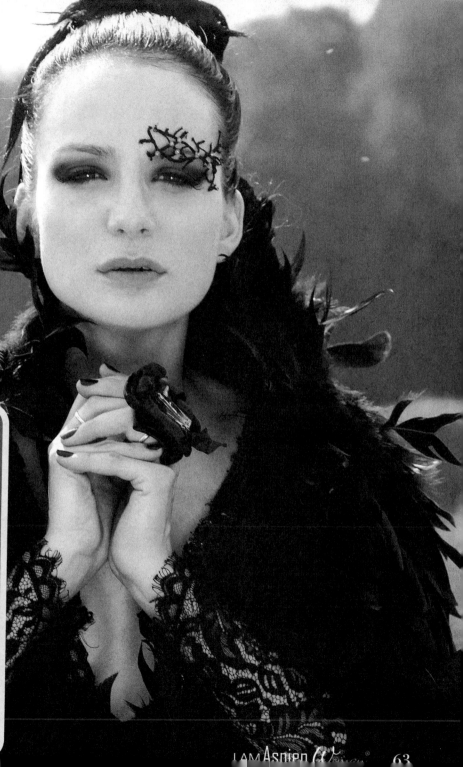

I am drawn to the unique, the different, the avant-garde. Everything else is like a grey, rainy winter's day: boring, dreary, unsatisfying ... I'm often told I take eccentric to a whole new level. I've always loved dressing differently, talking differently, anything different. It's who I am, I love my quirks but at times, other people look at me like I am a sideshow freak

It took many years for her to finally receive her diagnosis. It then took her six months to believe she was 2e (twice-exceptional), gifted with Autism (Asperger Syndrome). She had always thought she was dumb and we just thought she was eccentric. She found out why she processes information differently, why she struggles with disorganisation, socialising, communication, why she needs much more time to think and complete things and why she is such a fantastic singer, songwriter and musician.

— Family of late-diagnosed adult and successful musician

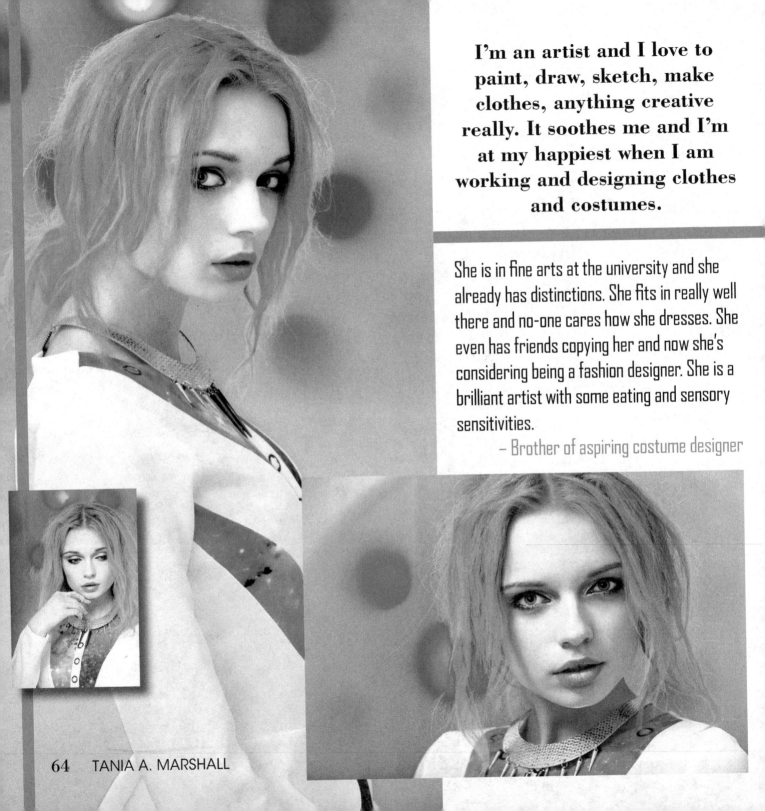

I'm an artist and I love to paint, draw, sketch, make clothes, anything creative really. It soothes me and I'm at my happiest when I am working and designing clothes and costumes.

She is in fine arts at the university and she already has distinctions. She fits in really well there and no-one cares how she dresses. She even has friends copying her and now she's considering being a fashion designer. She is a brilliant artist with some eating and sensory sensitivities.

– Brother of aspiring costume designer

Social

I'm not so good at staying in touch with my family or friends. I have had to learn to schedule in appointments to call my mum and family members. My brother installed a couple of apps on my devices that remind me to call them on their birthdays and I do have a Facebook account that my parents follow! I do not like chit-chat and my biggest challenge is by far stress and getting along with people. Social anxiety is crippling for me.

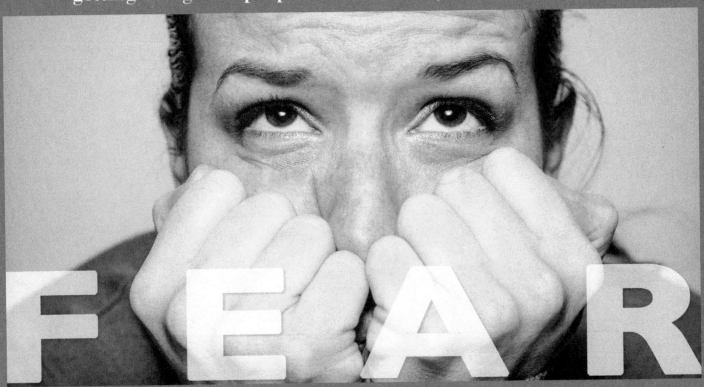

Females on the spectrum have varying degrees of difficulty with social interaction, social chit-chat, difficulty engaging in conversations (to them they have no purpose), understanding boundaries, levels of friendships and sometimes, a misguided sense of justice. Females with more severe difficulties struggle with the idea of the social hierarchy, in particular how to talk to or treat people of a different status, how to address conflict in a healthy way, how to be assertive (rather than passive or aggressive). Some have gotten into trouble for obsessing over and stalking people, meddling in affairs (due to feeling it is their business to police other people). This can get into trouble with bosses, teachers, church leaders, family members, the police, lawyers or other people in the community.

– Psychologist

I've worn so many masks, I don't even know who the 'real' me is. I can make eye contact and engage in chit-chat for a while; I have had ongoing self-esteem and identity issues and am now working with a professional who is helping me find out who I am and what my strengths are. No-one believes I have Asperger Syndrome.

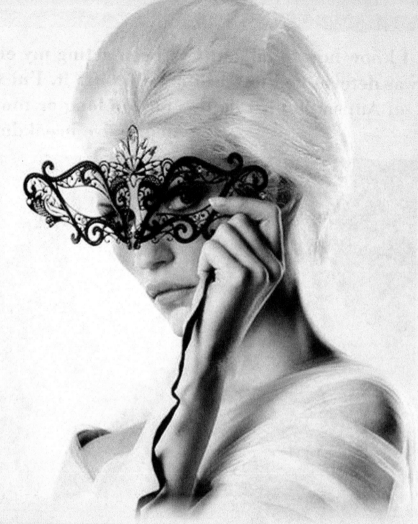

Model: Samantha Tomlin
Photography: Ardent Studios | www.Samanthatomlin.co.uk

The 'coping' strategies used by women are often referred to as 'masking' (learnt behaviours from observation and mimicking their peers) and can be a barrier to a diagnosis and accessing services. Many females have had years of developing a wide variety of coping mechanisms and strategies, and it is this practice that even enables some women to 'pass as normal' most of the time.

– Director of Autism Centre

I know how to fake it, I've been acting my entire life. It's exhausting but I was determined to teach myself to do it. I'm very good at masking my traits of Autism but if I do this for too long or too often it has led to me having depressive breakdowns.

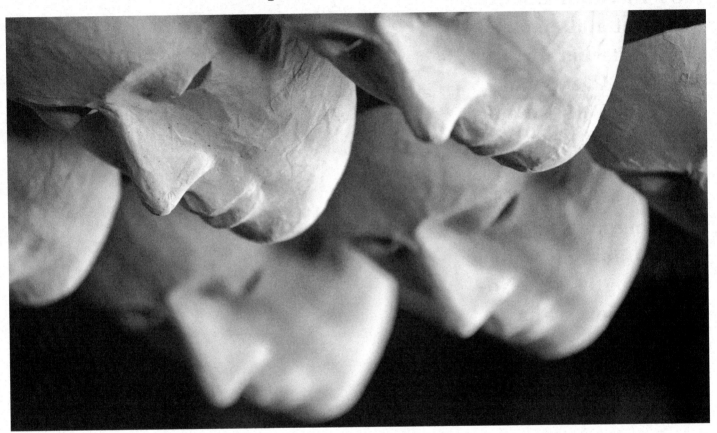

She has practised her whole life. Her use of social echolalia (copying, mimicking and acting) made it a challenge even for professionals not familiar with the unique female characteristics and traits. Many females can socialise quite well for short periods of time, make eye contact, do not have many repetitive behaviours. We struggled for years to understand her and often misunderstood her because we did not know nor had we heard of Autism or Asperger Syndrome back then.

– Mother of newly diagnosed daughter

Who am I? The Queen of Chameleons. Let's see … well, I started out as a Catholic schoolgirl tomboy, then a fashion star trying very hard to fit in, a corporate worker for an oil company, a Yogi in India for a year, then a punk rocker (yup, the whole Mohawk thing in every colour imaginable) who then turned into a love-and-peace-hippy-tattoo chick … and now? I'm at university getting my doctorate in philosophy! I can just about fit in anywhere.

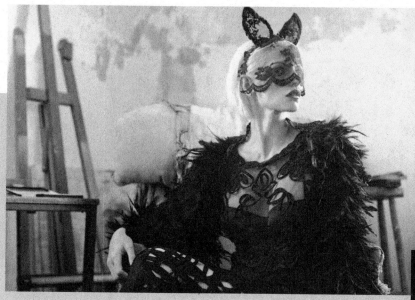

Model: Samantha Tomlin
Beachview Photograph

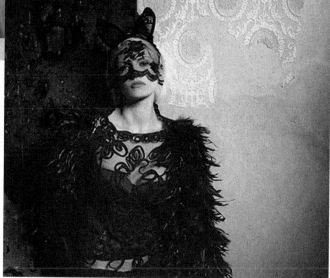

When we heard she was back in university we were somewhat relieved. We have worried about her for years … and years. We think she might have found herself now at 40, but she sure had us guessing what she was going to be doing next.

– Worried parents waiting to see
if daughter settles down

I use my intelligence and cognitive abilities to navigate through the social maze. I am confused about many things during a social encounter but I try hard to keep up and maintain appearances. I imagine how the conversations will go and I even have Plan B and plan C scripts ready just in case I need backup. Sometimes it still doesn't go according to plan. How come I didn't get the social handbook?

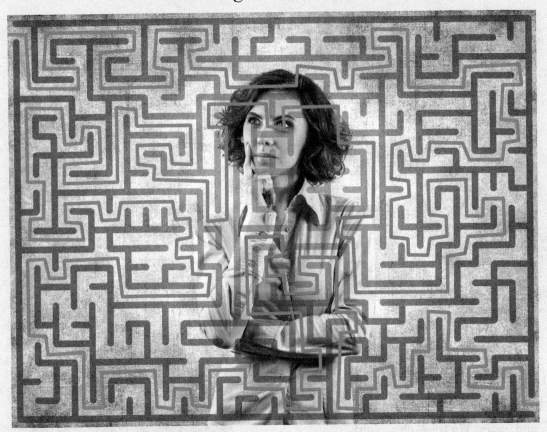

Life with late-diagnosed Autism is very hard on all of us as a family. The worst part for her is socially and then living independently. Socially, she overanalyses every part of her social interactions and can often be quite paranoid and highly anxious. She plans out the social interactions meticulously and often she will just disappear at a family gathering.
— Aunt of confused and socially anxious self-diagnosed female

I am a debater and I love to argue a point. I even argue for the sake of it! No matter how much I read and practise social skills, or non-verbal body language, I just can't get the nuances, the subtleties, never mind the complex expressions! I can't even keep up with myself (my own thoughts and opinions)! I feel like the mother alien ship dropped me off here from some other world and I'm just waiting to be picked up.

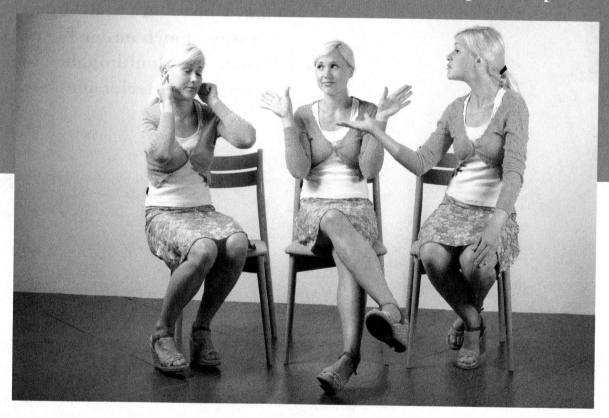

For her, faking it can take a lot of energy many times. She doesn't ever feel like she does it perfectly, even though she has studied and practised the right vocal tones, inflections, voice volume, verbal and non-verbal body language and facial expressions. She says she would rather do this than constantly struggle with not belonging anywhere. It was really important that people liked her; at times, far too important, that she would do almost anything to be liked.

– Foster mother of female desperate to fit in socially

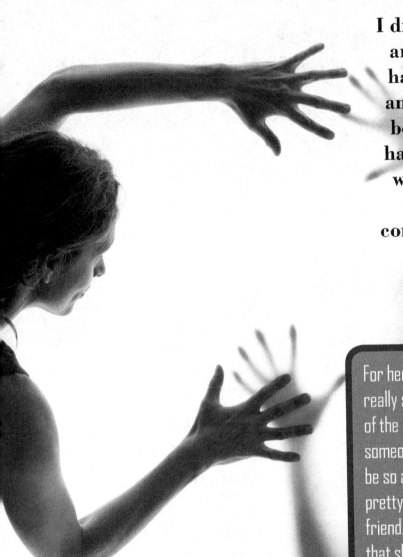

I did all kinds of stupid things to make and keep friends. I was desperate to have them and I would do just about anything. I joined a cult once, just to be accepted. I have not been able to have any kind of a relationship with a woman. I just don't know how. Guys are just so much easier for me to communicate with although sometimes they have ulterior motives.

For her, it's the reciprocal part of conversation that she really struggles with and she has also recently told me of the ongoing feeling that she's done something to upset someone but doesn't know what she did wrong. That must be so awful for her. This had led her to get into some pretty dangerous situations out of desperation to have a friend. She says she didn't understand she could say "no", that she could assert her boundaries, could or even dare to express herself. It didn't even occur to her that she could or should do so in some situations. It did not occur to her that she did not know how to do these things and we feel terrible. She has been taken advantage of many times.
– Mother of self-diagnosed daughter

I have a habit of getting into trouble socially with others and half the time I don't know what I've done wrong. This social communication thing is so hard. Why do I get in trouble for telling the truth?

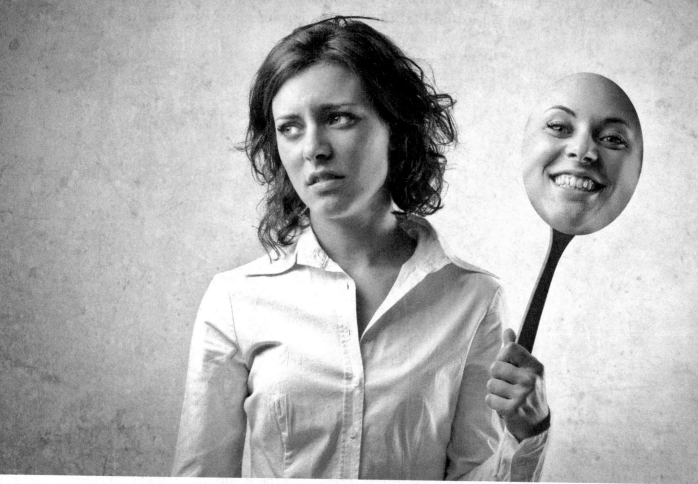

When she was younger she was way too emotionally honest and could not hide her feelings or emotions. She has learned to 'put on her face' when she goes to work. She lost a job once for answering honestly when her boss asked her if she was happy at work. She learned the hard way why sometimes we have to be socially 'untruthful'. She was right about all the things happening at work, but the unprofessional way she went about it and her lack of diplomacy got her fired. She is now on permanent disability.

– Parents of adult daughter living at home

I can socialise quite well … for small doses at a time … then I have a social hangover. When I was a child I was told that I would have a friend stay overnight, and Mum said when I'd filled my 'social cup', I would walk away and ask if they could go home. Of course, I don't do that anymore! I have always had social anxiety and I am much better one-on-one. I do find social chit-chat and the endless meetings challenging. I remember failing every group project when I was at university. They just sat around talking about nonsense and I wanted to get the work done.

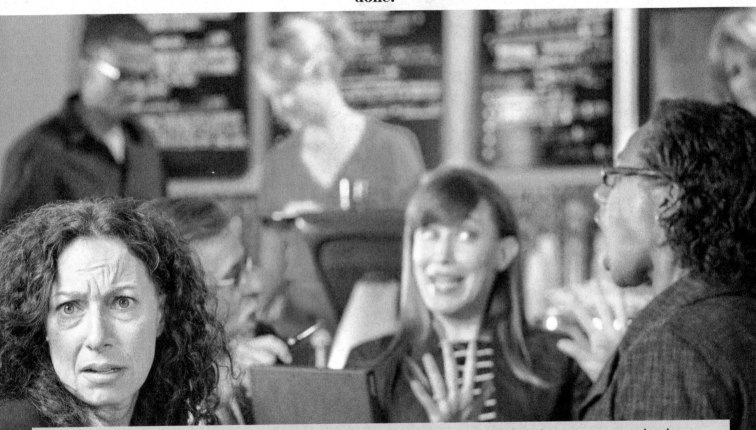

There exists a social spectrum that at one end a person may be so social that they cannot stand to be alone all the way to the other end (the person cannot tolerate being with people). When an individual learns where they are on the spectrum they can then make environmental and social adjustments. This can help with exhaustion and tiredness. Many individuals need 50% more downtime than the amount of time they spend socialising.

– Autism consultant

Education/Work

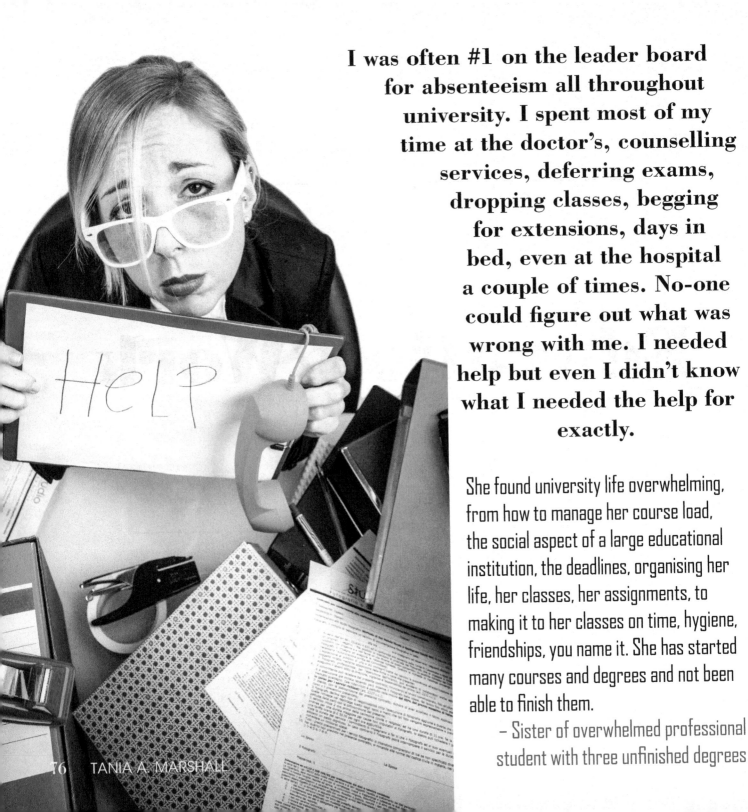

I was often #1 on the leader board for absenteeism all throughout university. I spent most of my time at the doctor's, counselling services, deferring exams, dropping classes, begging for extensions, days in bed, even at the hospital a couple of times. No-one could figure out what was wrong with me. I needed help but even I didn't know what I needed the help for exactly.

She found university life overwhelming, from how to manage her course load, the social aspect of a large educational institution, the deadlines, organising her life, her classes, her assignments, to making it to her classes on time, hygiene, friendships, you name it. She has started many courses and degrees and not been able to finish them.

– Sister of overwhelmed professional student with three unfinished degrees

I was studying for hours and hours and not remembering anything, so I went to the Learning Centre at my university and told them I thought there was something wrong with my brain. I had to do all these tests and found out I was smart and had some learning difficulties. They now allow me to write my exams in a quiet place, have extra time to complete my work and I don't have to take as many courses per semester.

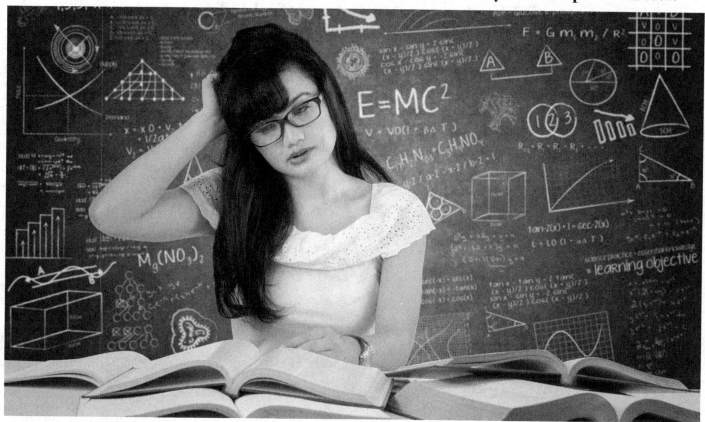

She started university at 16 years of age. She told me she got an A+, As and one B in her recent examinations, even though she studied the wrong subject for one of her exams! Even though she has a high IQ, she does have some learning difficulties. Some of the academic accommodations she receives are more time, permission to record the lectures and copies of all the PowerPoint presentations. They offered her sessions on learning organisational skills, time management, planning ahead, her learning and thinking style and how to study.

– Parents of teenage university student twice-exceptional daughter

I am intelligent and love learning about things I am interested in. I have a great long-term memory but I often can't remember my mother's birthday! I study ten times more than anybody else. My psychologist told me my brain processes like I'm on 'dial up' when everyone else is on Wi-Fi. No wonder I always feel behind.

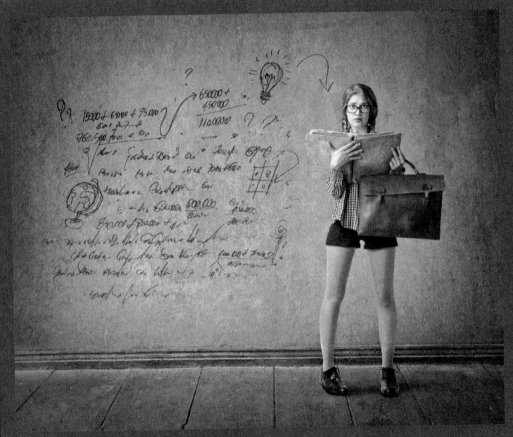

We created a joint project between Counselling Services and the Student Disability Services to facilitate the best learning environment for students with disabilities. We were seeing many smart females with a unique profile, These were grad students, many with scholarships, who were dropping out of courses, missing semesters, constantly getting deferrals, extensions, having nervous breakdowns. We were provided with some in-service training on Asperger Syndrome and the presenter spoke about female Autism. We now have a support group for Autistic females, free assessment, diagnosis, learning profiling and academic accommodations and support here at the university.

– Director

I am a lifelong learner. I started here as an undergraduate student and have just got my second PhD. I crave knowledge and need to know the answer to everything. Now I have a daughter who is the same. It is only now that I know how much I must have driven my mother crazy with my constant questioning. I love the university culture and lifestyle. I feel like I really fit in here.

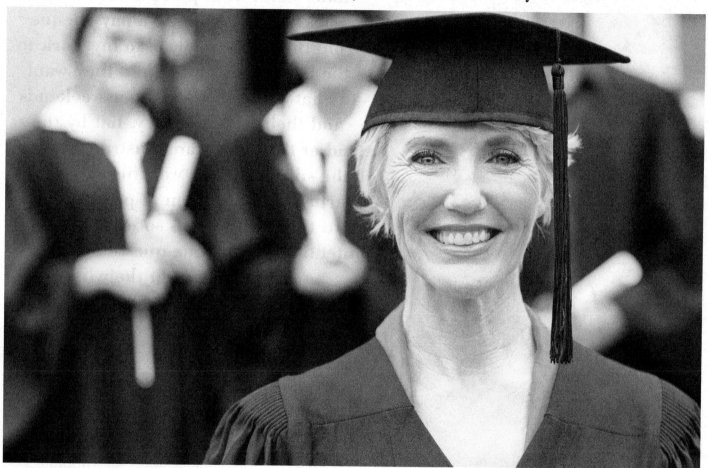

My mum has 'weirdo intellect'. She's ok with me saying that. I mean, she has two PhDs. I mean, who does that?! We thought it was amazing when she got her first one! We asked her, "Why?" She said, "Because I can." Do we call her like 'Doctor Doctor' now?

– Nine-year-old daughter of professor (of lifelong learning)

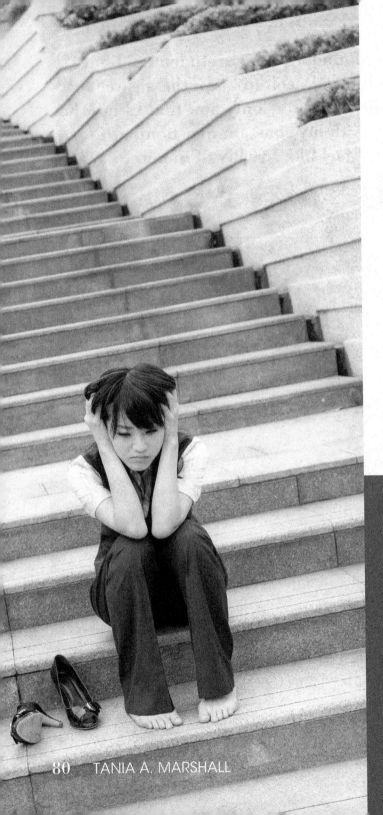

I excel at my job, getting continual promotions, but it's the communicating with co-workers who want to be chatty that I find a real challenge. I can't understand what place chatter has at work? I am accepting a pay cheque from them and want to do my work to the best of my ability and they want to chat with me about their weekends and their kids? I do try, but by the end of the week I am frustrated by all the silliness. I am working on being warm and more open to people. I like to think in systems so what I do is intentionally ask one question a day to a co-worker about their life.

She has had many different jobs, none have been long-term. She was really struggling in the work environment and not knowing why. She has taken many sick days, not showed up to work or just walked out. She would talk to me about watching the other people at work and seeing them making friends and bonding and talking personal stuff, and just be in total wonderment of how it all works and how they do it without even thinking about it.

– Parents of young woman trying to find the right fit

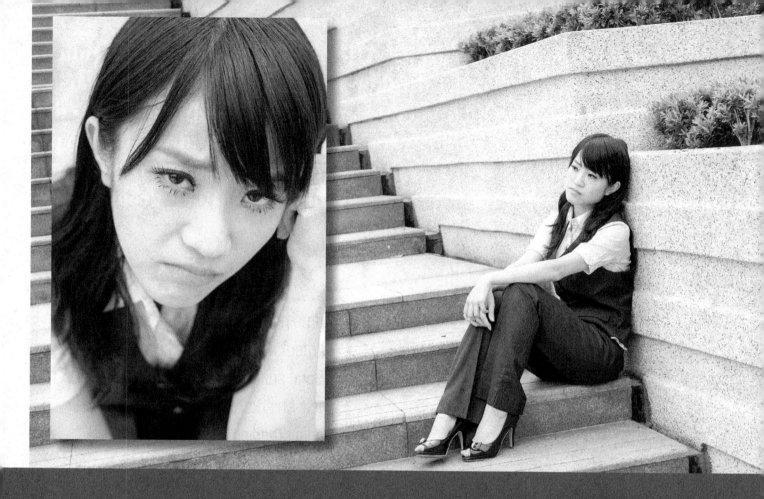

It has taken her years to find the right work environment. She worked in a busy call centre once; it was an insane place of sensory overload, multitasking, noise, fluorescent lighting, and too many people all speaking at once. She also had created her social scripts to use at work but when they changed it, she had no backup plan and that would upset her and usually lead her to getting into some kind of trouble.

– Autism employment specialist

I called time-out on my career. After my diagnosis, I took time to learn about what type of thinker I am, what my strengths are, what kind of environment I needed and what I really wanted to do. Learning about my strengths, what I am good at and the best type of work environment was the launch I needed to then start my own business. I am my own boss and self-employment is a great fit for me.

Some females struggle through life without knowing what they are good at and some seem to naturally fall into their strengths. Once females have an understanding of the way they think and experience the world, then explore, nurture and start focusing on their strengths, they can be unstoppable. I just met a middle-aged self-diagnosed woman who only recently started painting (self-taught) and already people are wanting to buy her art.

– Psychologist

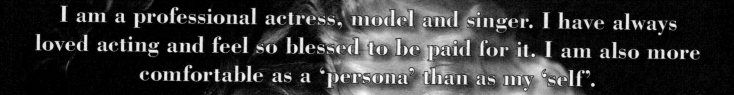

I am a professional actress, model and singer. I have always loved acting and feel so blessed to be paid for it. I am also more comfortable as a 'persona' than as my 'self'.

She was born to act. From a very early age she took on the roles of the teacher, the principal, the doctor, the director. She would 'boss' her teddy bears around, directing them and telling them what to do.

– Sister of professional actress

I am a professional singer and songwriter. I have been singing and dancing since I was four years of age. I was an X-factor finalist and now have a recording contract. I sing opera too. I remember driving my sister nearly mad by singing the same notes and bits of songs over and over. My biggest challenge is being watched when I perform. I hate it.

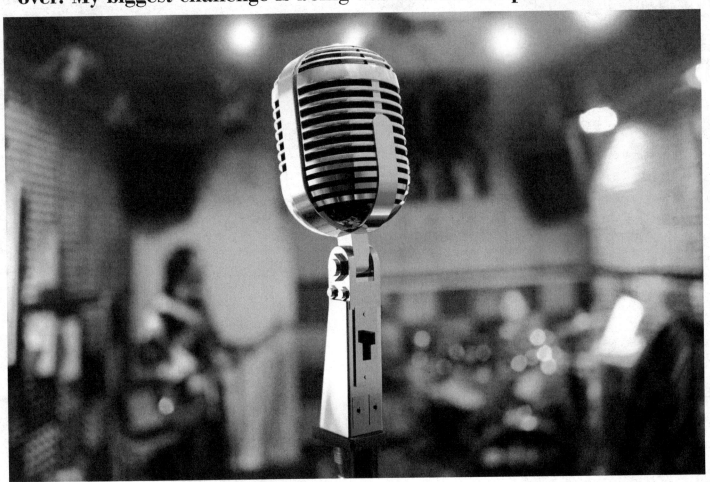

She was born with perfect pitch and loves to sing. She does struggle from time to time with paralysing panic attacks that can prevent her from performing in front of others. She is working on this with a psychologist.
– Proud parents of gifted singer with Asperger Syndrome

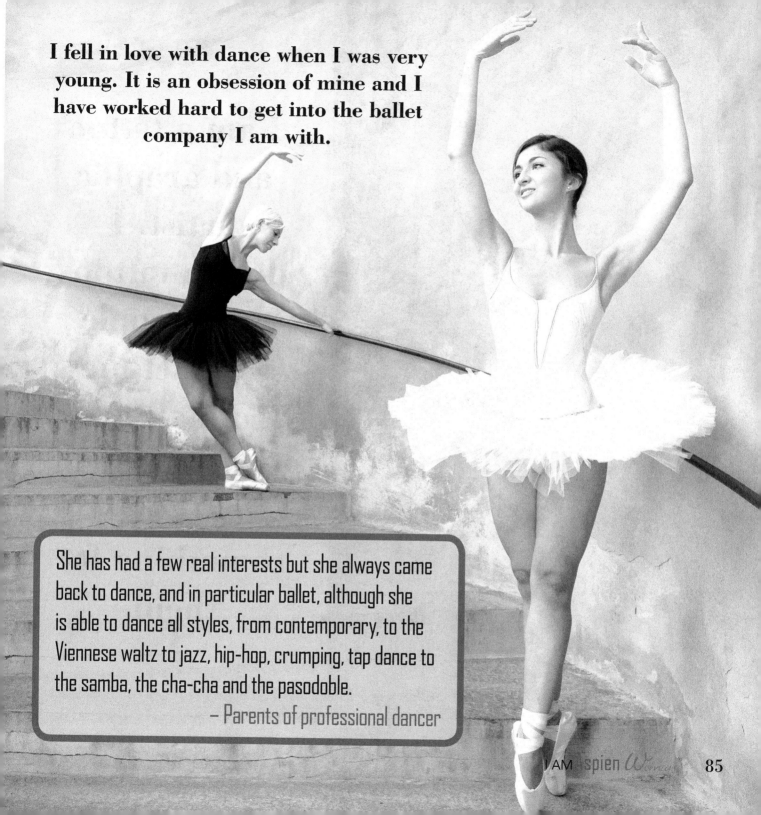

I fell in love with dance when I was very young. It is an obsession of mine and I have worked hard to get into the ballet company I am with.

She has had a few real interests but she always came back to dance, and in particular ballet, although she is able to dance all styles, from contemporary, to the Viennese waltz to jazz, hip-hop, crumping, tap dance to the samba, the cha-cha and the pasodoble.

– Parents of professional dancer

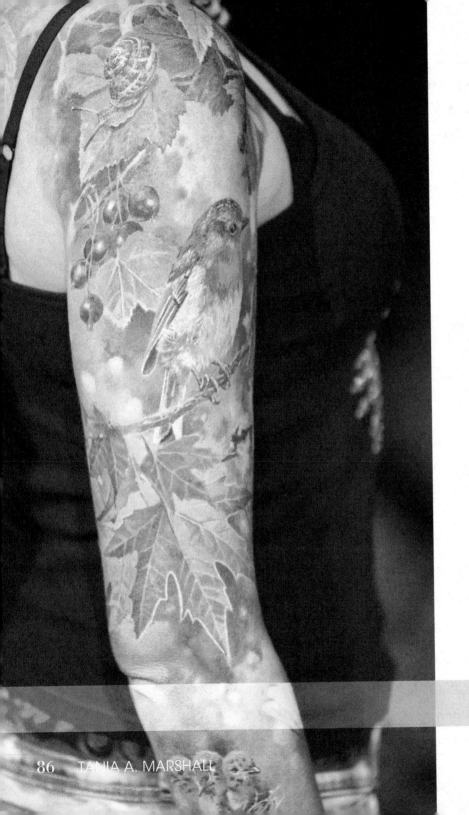

I am a tattoo
and graphic
artist. I
design tattoos
and people
contact me
from all over
the country
to design
something for
them.

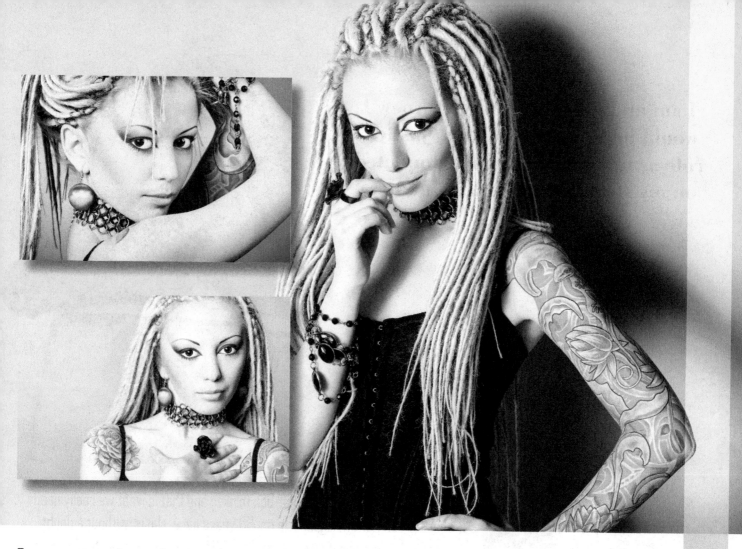

From very early on she was drawing, doodling and sketching. As a teenager, one of her friends asked if he could use one of her sketches for his first tattoo. This was the impetus for her career. She is very popular.

— Mother of young tattoo artist and AspienWoman

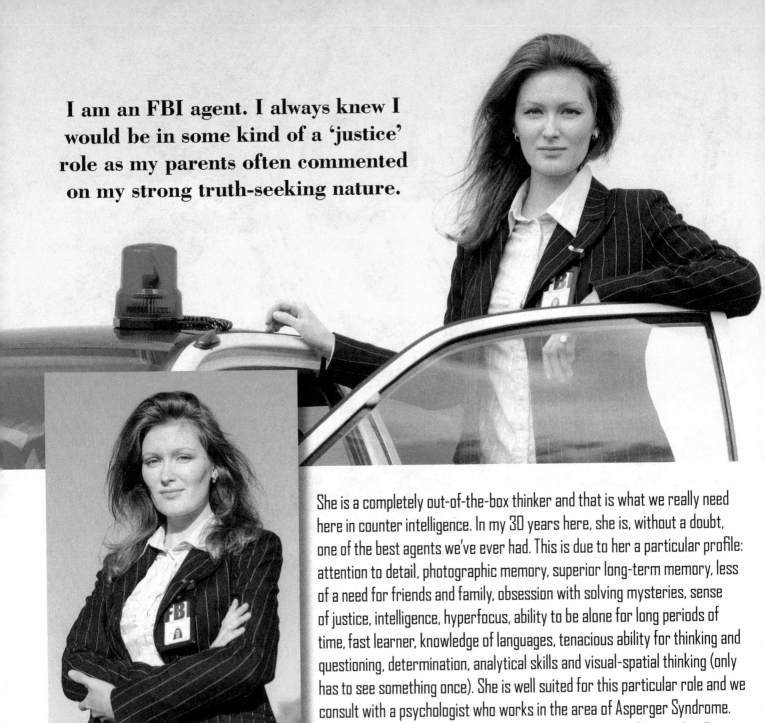

I am an FBI agent. I always knew I would be in some kind of a 'justice' role as my parents often commented on my strong truth-seeking nature.

She is a completely out-of-the-box thinker and that is what we really need here in counter intelligence. In my 30 years here, she is, without a doubt, one of the best agents we've ever had. This is due to her a particular profile: attention to detail, photographic memory, superior long-term memory, less of a need for friends and family, obsession with solving mysteries, sense of justice, intelligence, hyperfocus, ability to be alone for long periods of time, fast learner, knowledge of languages, tenacious ability for thinking and questioning, determination, analytical skills and visual-spatial thinking (only has to see something once). She is well suited for this particular role and we consult with a psychologist who works in the area of Asperger Syndrome.

– Director, Counter Intelligence

I was one of the first female pilots in my country. I loved the freedom of flying and being by myself. Although that was a long time ago, I still marvel about the invention of the plane and how far they have come.

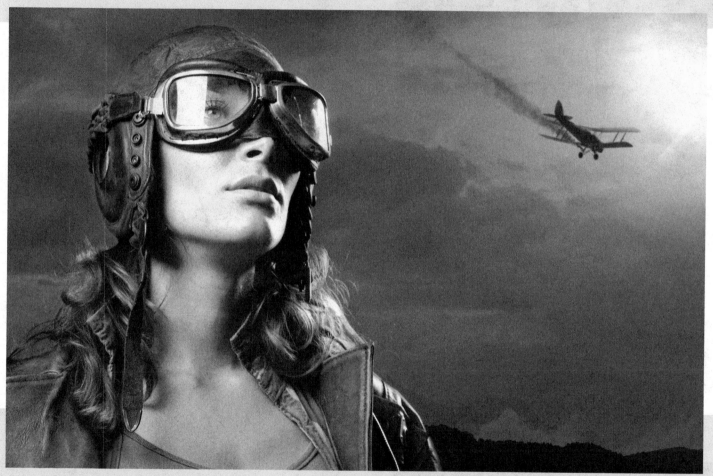

Grandma has the coolest stories about her plane and flying and the places she went, and even a couple of near crashes! She is so cool!

– Young grandson who wants to fly planes

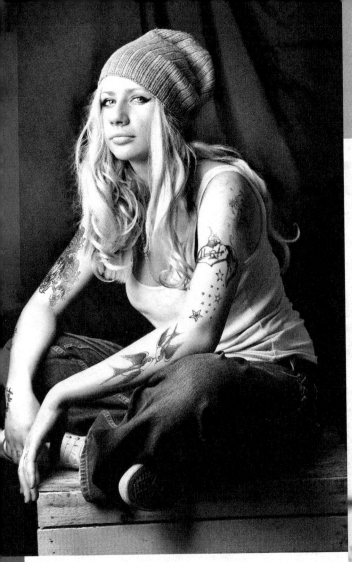

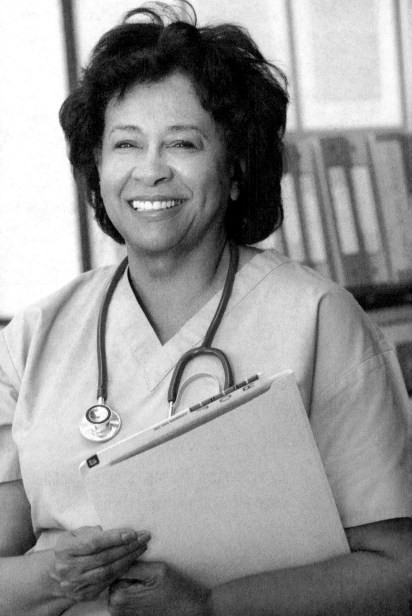

I work in the helping profession. I am a social worker and I work at a day shelter for homeless people.

I am a nurse working in emergency mental health. I am good in crisis situations.

TANIA A. MARSHALL

I am a psychiatrist and I love understanding and helping others.

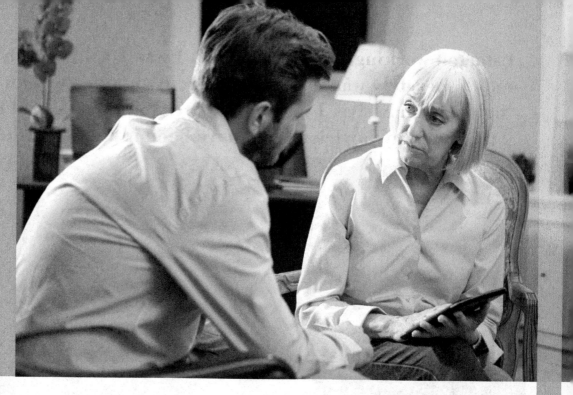

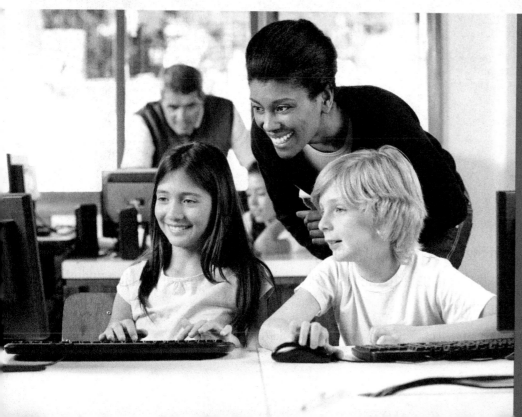

I have always gravitated towards children and teaching. I am now a special needs teacher working with children with Autism and it is very fulfilling for me.

I started working in this area when I was 16. I had run away from home and desperately wanted some peace. My mother was an alcoholic and my father was abusive. I moved to the city and just could not keep a job. I then met my boyfriend and have been in the sex industry ever since.

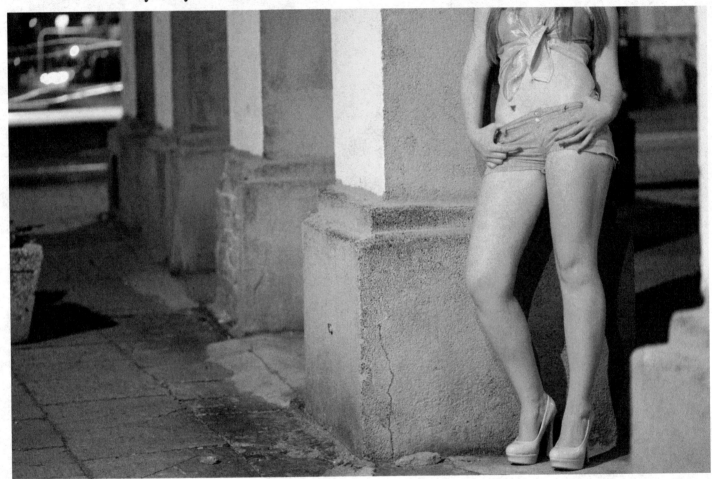

A proportion of females working in the sex trade have Asperger Syndrome or Autism. They are at higher risk for becoming sex trade workers due in part to their social naivety, living in poverty, drug addictions and challenges with finding and keeping work.

– Social worker who works with street workers

Sensory Sensitivities

I have auditory processing challenges. I often don't catch what is said and I'm always asking people to repeat themselves. People whispering in a lecture would drive me crazy and I'd have to get up and move somewhere else!

She is highly sensitive. She dislikes fireworks, balloons popping, vacuums, and too many people talking. She would say the noise hurts her and makes her feel sick. She hears things more loudly, sees things more clearly and feels things much more than others do. She also can hear what everybody is saying in the house, so we really have to watch what we say!

– Siblings of highly sensitive person

I learned about my unique sensory profile from my psychologist. This helped me to understand all eight senses, whether I was a 'seeker' or an 'avoider' and helped me create a sensory management kit. My kit has ear phones, my Beatz headphones (a noise cancellation feature), Irlen glasses, scarf, hat, stress ball, fiddle beads and my lavender necklace. It goes with me everywhere. My headphones really help my misophonia (hatred of sound).

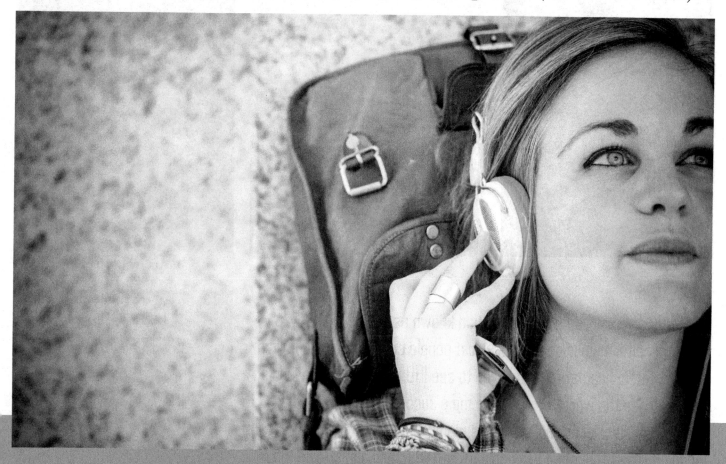

Each client I support works with me individually on understanding their unique sensory profile and creating a sensory management kit, as part of making unique, individual environmental modifications to assist them in day-to-day functioning.
— Psychologist, Tania A. Marshall

My Autism gives me a multicoloured world ... I am a self-taught artist. My art is usually inspired by how I feel more than anything I really look at ...

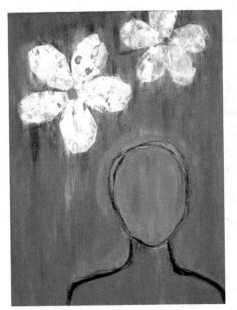

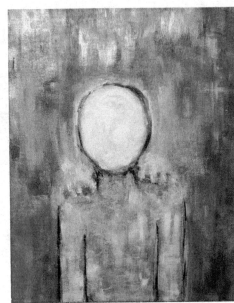

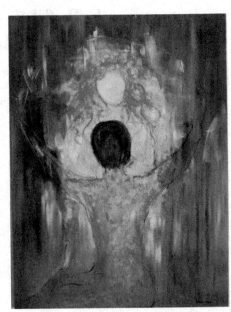

Art by Lexington Sherbin

I recently discovered I have a condition known as tetrachromacy, a fourth cone for colour perception. Most people can see about a million colours. Tetrachromats are believed to see 100 million! I love my vision and how I see the world. It has made me a successful artist ... what you see as grey sky or rocks I see as magical colours of pinks, greens and blues. I just found out I see colours other people cannot see. How cool is that? I thought everybody could see what I see.

– Successful artist with formal diagnosis of Autism Spectrum Condition

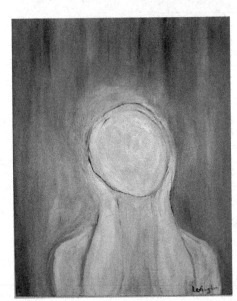

I am a musician. I have a type of synaesthesia. I literally see sounds in front of me which helps me know where to sing, for example. It makes me a better musician. I see sounds as dots and lines right in front of me (Maja Nillson, Musician and Song Writer).

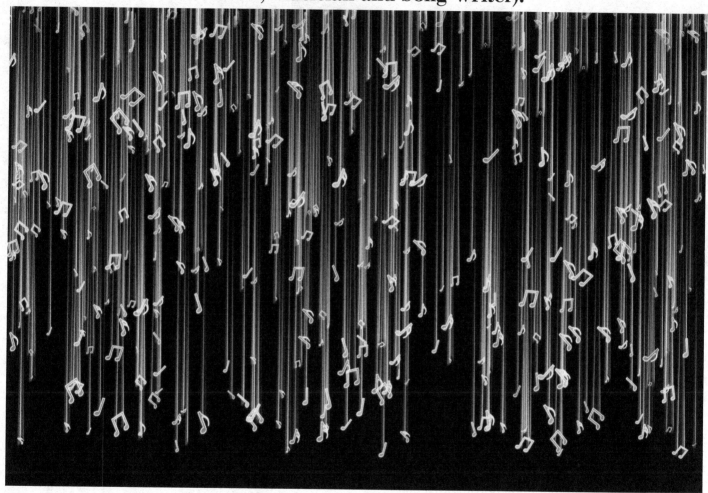

Synaesthesia is a neurological condition where stimulation of one sensory or cognitive pathway leads to automatic, involuntary experiences in a second sensory or cognitive pathway. There are many different types of synaesthesia and we are learning about new ones all the time.

– Neuroscientist and Autism researcher

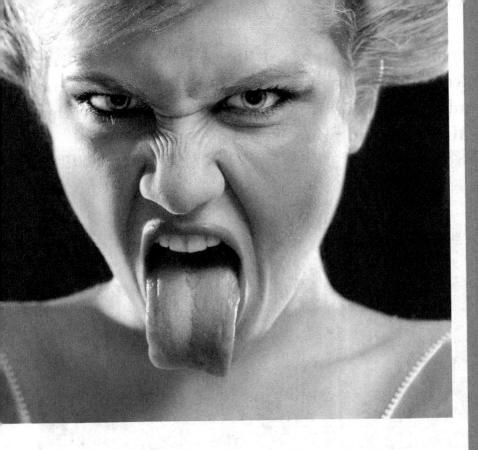

She has always been sensitive. Years ago, they told us she was an attention seeker and it was all because of our parenting, but we didn't give up until we found someone who listened to us. One of the first things the psychologist gave us was a 'sensory assessment'. It was *then* that we understood just how real her complaints are.

– Parents with a new understanding of adult daughter with sensory processing issues

My sensory issues are frustrating for me. I can only eat bland food because anything else tastes so spicy and fizzy drinks feel like my tongue is burning off! I've always had a problem swallowing tablets. My mother used to crush any tablets I had to have and give them to me with a teaspoon of honey. I can swallow small tablets with water now but larger ones have to be broken, dissolved or crushed.

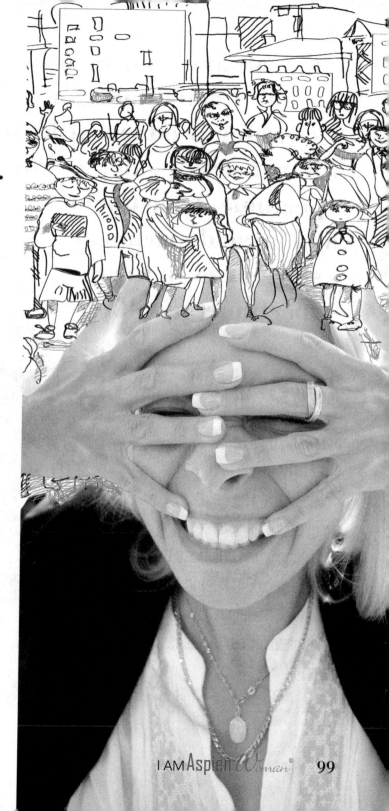

Ever since I was young I have been intuitive; my emotional empathy is hyperactive! I strongly *feel* other people's pain. It can be overwhelming, especially in crowds. I never talk about it because it is way too far 'out there', that never mind others, but to me, it sounds crazy. I don't know how I know but I just *feel* other people's feelings. I know when people are lying to me. I can *feel* it. It's a different way of knowing for me and I have had to work hard to learn how to use it.

She has a tendency to forget she is watching a film or television. It's almost like she is 'inside the story', then once it's finished, she needs time to transition from the movie to present-day reality. She has never been able to watch violence, sex, conflict or horror-type movies. She can't be around people much. She says she can feel their pain like it's happening to her. They told us that she could have schizophrenia but it doesn't really fit. Then we heard about mirror-touch synaesthesia and had a light bulb moment!

– Father of highly sensitive hermit

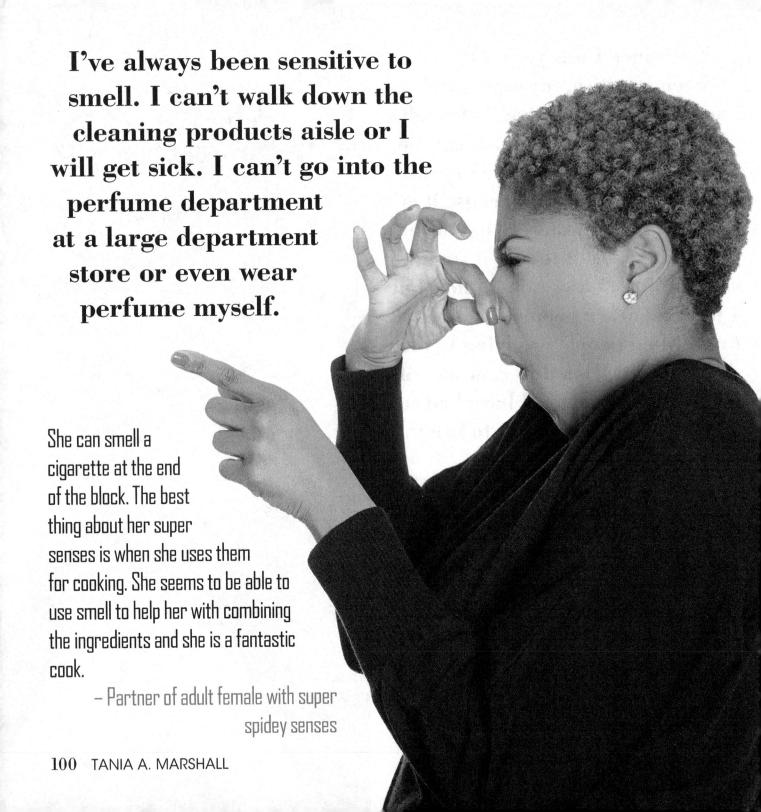

I've always been sensitive to smell. I can't walk down the cleaning products aisle or I will get sick. I can't go into the perfume department at a large department store or even wear perfume myself.

She can smell a cigarette at the end of the block. The best thing about her super senses is when she uses them for cooking. She seems to be able to use smell to help her with combining the ingredients and she is a fantastic cook.

– Partner of adult female with super spidey senses

I knock into things all the time, fall over sometimes, have bruises all over me, spill food or drink on my shirt, I miss my mouth … it's frustrating and embarrassing at times when I lose my balance.

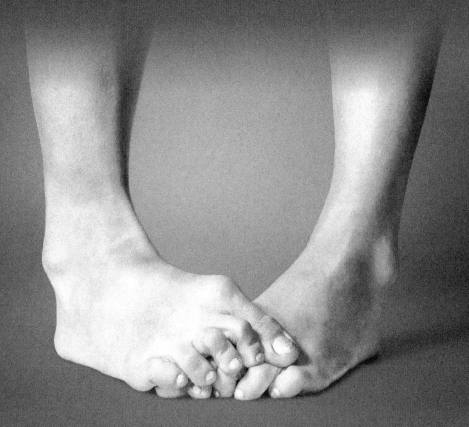

Our daughter can fall out of a chair she's sitting in, knock into objects and trip out the doorway, all whilst answering the doorbell! She has always had difficulty with coordination issues.
— Parents of clumsy adult female with impeccable fine motor skills

I have never liked to be hugged and I can't stand light touch. I really like deep pressure and weighted blankets though.

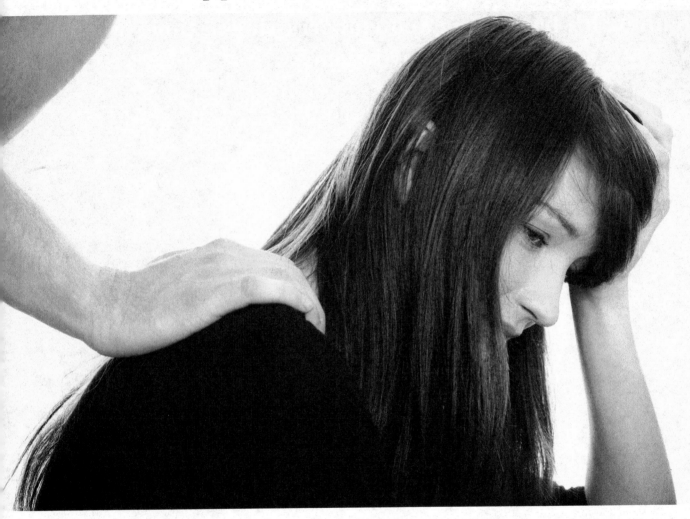

We always took offence when she recoiled if we hugged her. Now we know it's not because she doesn't love us. It's because to her it hurts. Sensory experiences often upset and overwhelm her. She doesn't like her food touching and still has noise issues, although overall we would say her sensory issues have improved somewhat since her childhood. We now just place our hand firmly on her shoulder and she really likes this.

– Parents of AspienWoman

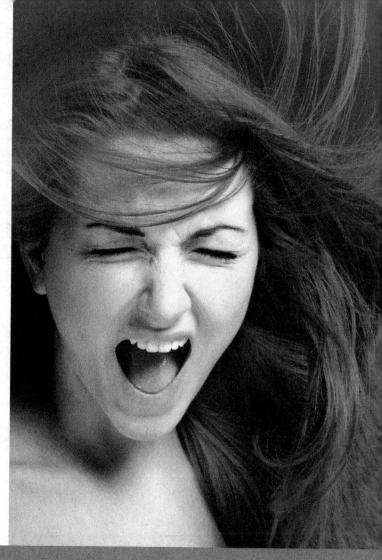

I am prone to meltdowns and I can't control them. They happen when I'm overloaded or overwhelmed. It's so embarrassing and I tend to feel ashamed about my behaviour afterwards. Then I don't know how to fix it and it looks like to others that I just don't care. I work so hard to pretend to be normal at work and school, but when I get home I explode.

Socially speaking, from very early on she has catastrophised and misinterpreted other people's intentions. There have been times where we have no idea how she came to her conclusions about another person, friendship or work relationship. She has burnt bridges on more than one occasion and can be very socially inappropriate.

– Cousin of socially awkward adult stumbling through life without the book of unwritten social rules

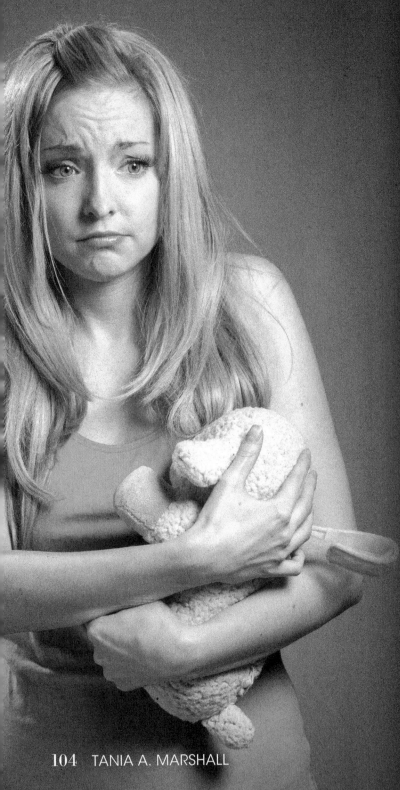

I do certain things over and over again. I fidget, twirl my hair, leg-bounce, rub or massage my feet together. I'm usually always doing something with my hands whether it is biting my nails or skin, picking at my skins, chewing my hair, fidgeting with something. I grind my teeth and bite the inside of my mouth. I also sway when I'm standing up. I was in trouble for constantly leg bouncing when I was at work because it distracted others. I just learnt its called self-regulation or self-soothing.

She has a few sensory issues. She needs a highly controlled environment to sleep in: ear plugs, white noise, fan on even if it's freezing, heavy blankets, complete darkness. She loves the feeling because it's soothing and helps her sleep. Repetitive, loud and high-pitched noises and certain textures are painful for her.

— Father determined to understand his highly anxious daughter

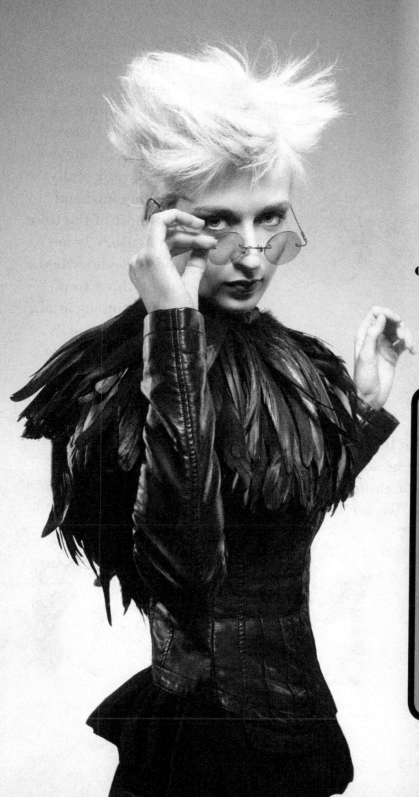

I have difficulty processing visual information and didn't discover I had Irlen Syndrome until I was 40. I don't just wear them to look cool. Having my glasses has really help me see better. I had constant headaches. I couldn't read properly. Life is a lot easier looking through my blue lenses.

She has always had problems with fluorescent or bright lighting, the sun or flashing lights. She said to us she felt like her eyes were on fire. We had her eyes checked a number of times over the years and found nothing. She would complain about the words moving on the paper and not being able to remember what she was reading. She works in the fashion media industry now and is known as the 'model with the cool glasses'. They love her.
– Grandmother of fashion model

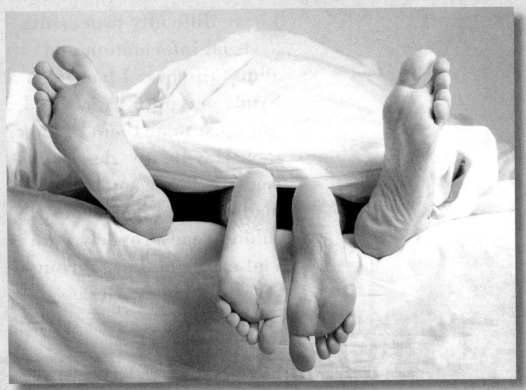

I'm one of many who experience disengagement due to overwhelming sensory feelings. At times I cannot tolerate even cuddling. I really love my husband but most of the time my sensory issues made me horrified at anything to do with intimacy at all. I was so sensorily overwhelmed that not only would I get a headache, but the sheets scratched my skin, the candles he put on stunk to high heaven, the music was too loud, his beard scratched me and my husband felt like he was always having to coerce me into it. He thought I didn't love him and was just making excuses because I told him I didn't like the colours and the smell in the room. We are headed for divorce, so we agreed to see a clinical sexologist.

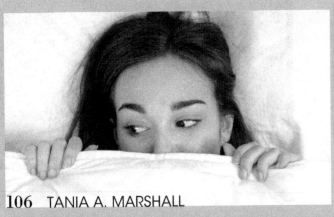

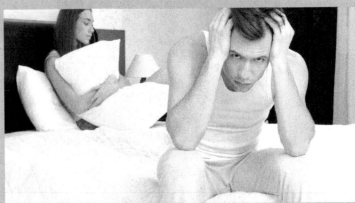

We found out I have 'adult sexual-sensory dysfunction' or ASSD. We learnt the ways in which sensory information is processed and how it can have an unrecognised and direct impact on the quality of an individual's or couple's sex life. As a child I was aversive to certain types of touch. In particular, gentle stroking drove me crazy but I always enjoyed firm, non-moving pressure. Even certain types of fabric, like certain types of sheets, turned out to be a factor in interfering with our private lives. We were asked to make a list of triggers, reactions and situations that we thought disrupted our sex life. In our sessions we learnt to make modifications and other strategies which have made us much happier. Few professionals exist who understand the connection between sensory processing sensitivities and sexual difficulties.

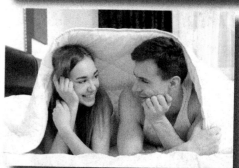

– A much happier couple

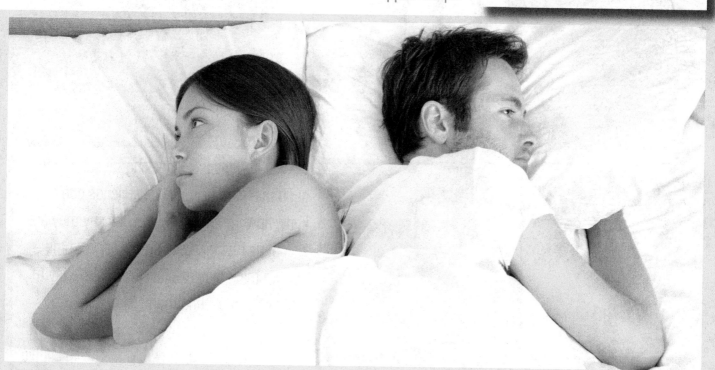

I am a super-senser who seeks touch. I have always been sensitive all over. So for instance, my husband just caresses my side or kisses me and it transports me to a whole other world. I'm very lucky he is similar to me.

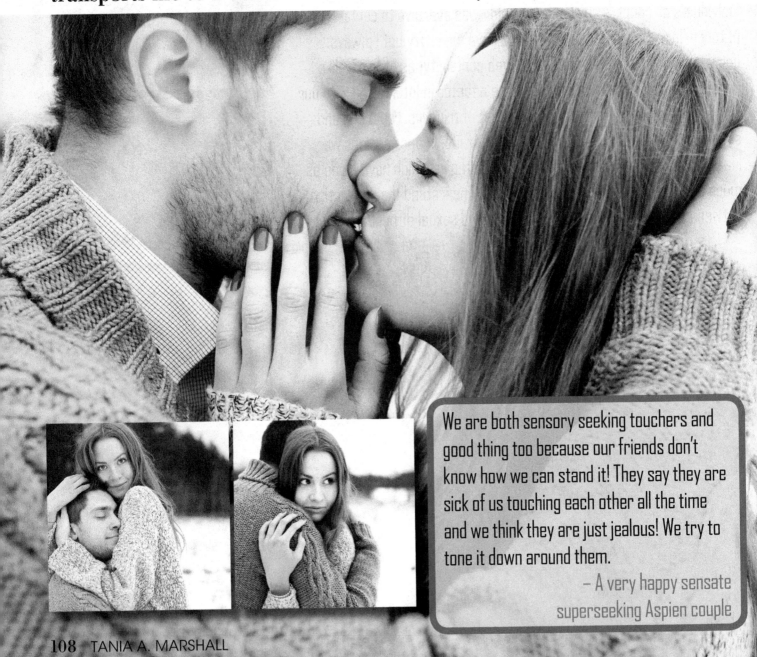

We are both sensory seeking touchers and good thing too because our friends don't know how we can stand it! They say they are sick of us touching each other all the time and we think they are just jealous! We try to tone it down around them.

– A very happy sensate superseeking Aspien couple

Emotional

I worry … a lot. I worry about worrying! I have plenty of fears that have changed over the years. I have had panic attacks over death, thinking about giving birth, attending highly important events, moving, being watched, any kind of change and lots of negative 'what if' thinking.

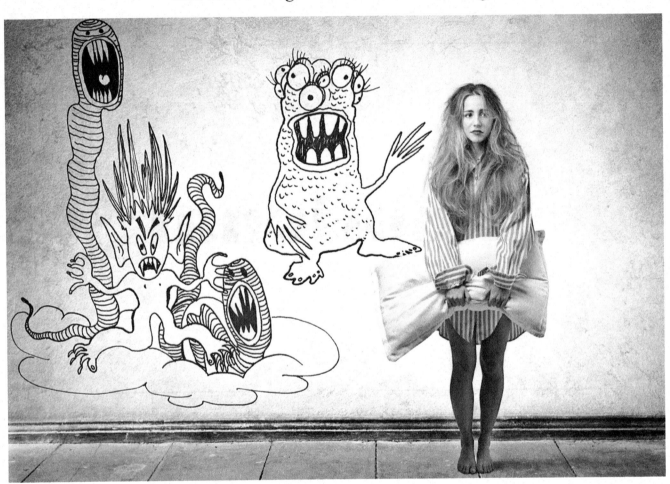

As a highly visual thinker and mirror-touch synaesthate, she is highly distressed by visual images or television that depicts animal abuse, abuse to children and the news. She is unable to remove the pictures from her brain and is highly disturbed by them. She has never watched a horror or scary movie. We used to have to monitor what she watched and read. The images haunt her for ages. She is just unable to cope with those aspects of the world.

– Mother of highly sensitive 'worrier' daughter

I have struggled emotionally my whole life. Stress and anxiety are my Kryptonite. It is that I feel TOO much, and feel it most of the time. I have strong emotions and have difficulty managing them.

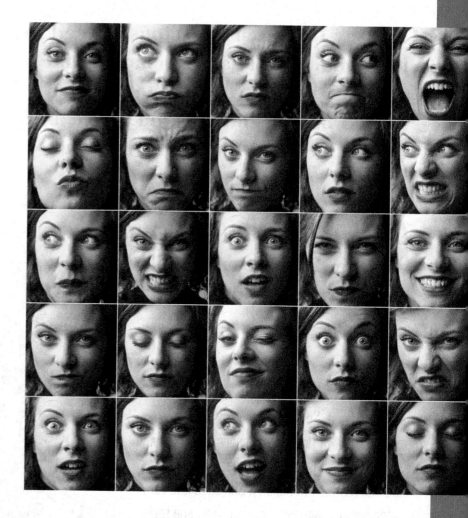

She was born with a frown on her face. I was often telling her to smile and she would say, "What for?" and I would say, "To be friendly". She is still as serious now as she was back then.
– Mother of emotional and serious daughter

They say I'm intense, serious, I need to lighten up ... they say, "You look angry, you have to change that face." I say, "I'm not angry." They say, "Yes, but you look angry." I say, "I'm concentrating on music and thinking." They think I'm in a bad mood. I'm not angry; I'm just a person who thinks a lot. They call it 'Resting Bitchy Face' on YouTube. It made a whole lot of sense when I watched it.

Her facial expressions have always been just slightly different. Sometimes she stares too much and most of time she appears to be worried or very intense. She often clenches her jaw and grinds her teeth from anxiety. She says it is very hard for her to make her face look how she feels on the inside and that she really has to work hard at it. She also mentioned the other day about having to work on her tone of voice. My, that must be exhausting for her!
– Grandmother of recently diagnosed daughter with high-functioning Autism

I have struggled for years with managing stress, my emotions and my thoughts. My psychologist helped me to make changes to maintain both an internally and externally calm environment. I am learning not to be so hard on myself and to practise extreme self-care.

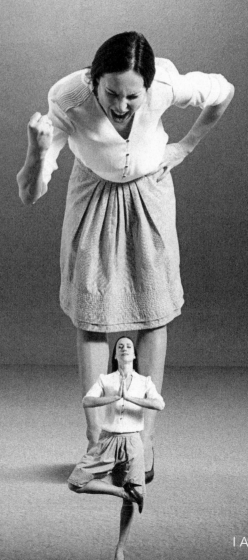

She is prone to 'depressive attacks' and her brain appears to be wired to be a half glass empty. She is learning how to be happy and rewire her brain by changing her thoughts. She is determined to beat her 'stinkin thinkin', as she calls it, and has been working very hard on her thoughts and her feelings in her sessions. We are noticing a difference.

– Family of AspienMother, learning and practising how to think in more helpful ways

I have learnt that whenever I'm uncomfortable or anxious I tend to avoid demands, those situations or tasks. I can become so overwhelmed by the enormousness of a task or the group or the situation. It wasn't that I couldn't do the task. I just didn't know where to start and I would get lost in amongst all of the steps or the follow-up of a task. I still do this at times but I have had help from a professional and I have done a lot of personal work in this area of my life, including using many strategies that I have recently learned.

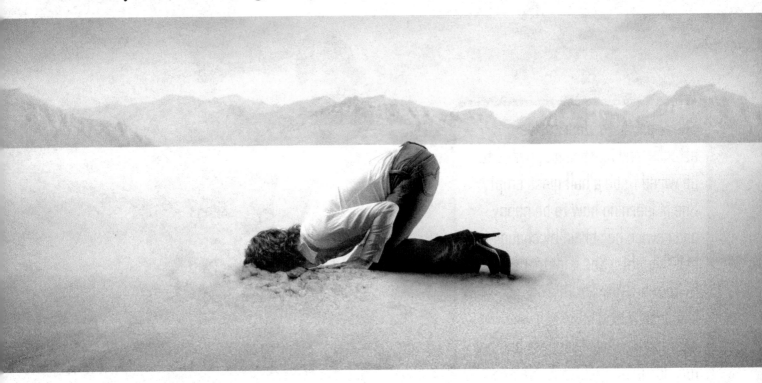

When she was younger, if she didn't like a situation or didn't want to do something she would just pretend it wasn't happening, or make up all kinds of outlandish excuses on why she couldn't do something, rather than confront it and deal with the issue. She can avoid demands that overwhelm her, make her highly anxious, if she feels the task is too big or she might think that she cannot achieve a particular goal or it's not going to be perfect.

– Parents of perfectionist learning to face demands and problem solve

My doctor recently told me I have Chronic Fatigue Syndrome, my stress was too high and my adrenals are exhausted. The corporate world is just not a good fit for me and I am now on medical leave. I recently saw a psychiatrist who suggested I have some traits of Autism and referred me for an adult female assessment.

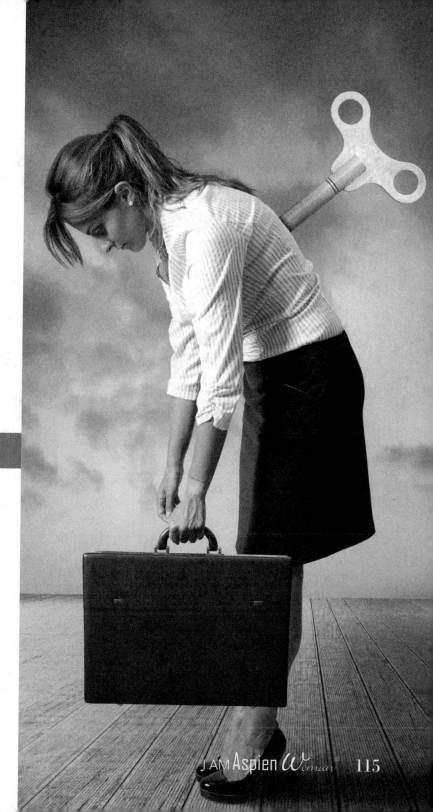

She is considering leaving the corporate world. She is fantastic at what she does and makes great money. She is an executive manager and has to attend numerous all-day meetings that frustrate her enormously. She manages over 100 employees and loves this part of her work, but has challenges with her senior managers, weekly meetings, chit-chat and conflict resolution.

– Sister of energy depleted and exhausted corporate employee

I feel like I am allergic to stress. For as long as I can remember, I've always been stressed, anxious or angry. It has been my #1 issue. I went for a massage once and she said I was the tensest person she had ever met. I have adrenal fatigue now.

Sometimes we feel like we are living with two different people, Jekyll and Hyde. She comes home very stressed and irritable.
– Family of stressed-out mother who now loves her relaxation training classes

I have challenges with anger. It just overtakes me at times and I cannot control it. I have had some spectacular meltdowns and even ended up in hospital once. I just could not cope at all with life and the pressures and responsibilities of it all. I feel like I'm always in the extreme; I don't feel anything in between the extremes.

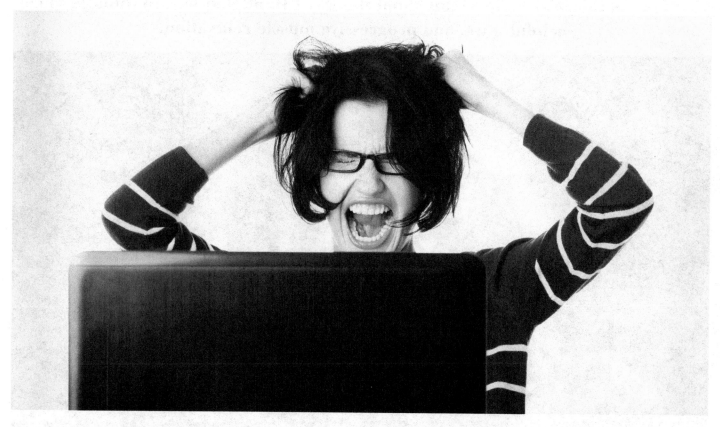

Anger, anxiety and the inability to manage stress and communicate effectively can ruin many friendships, work relationships, jobs and families. A large part of my job entails supporting people with Autism through change, teaching life skills, assertive training, modified cognitive behavioural therapy techniques, communication skills and perspective taking.

– Social worker and family therapist

I have found it helpful to learn about my 'stress dial', levels of stress, the ways my body tells me I'm stressed and the situations that stress me out. A comprehensive extreme self-care program has really helped me to feel calmer and more in control of my emotions. My program includes medication, physical exercise, meditation and solitude, a modified Cognitive Behavioural Behaviour program, distress tolerance work, learning about the way I think and how to think in more helpful ways, and progressive muscle relaxation.

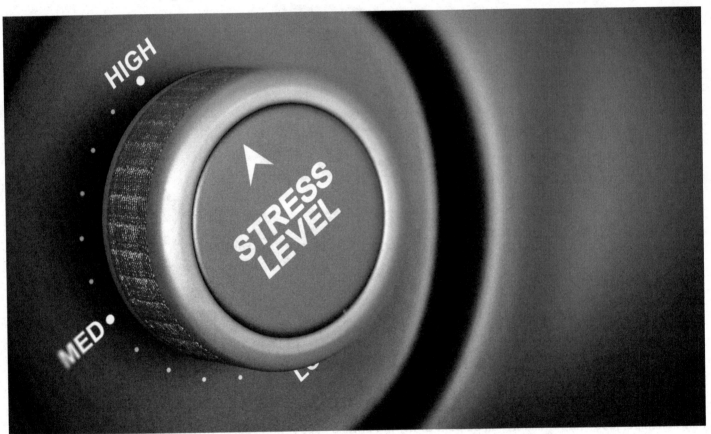

When I inquired as to why, she reported that she didn't like the feelings of "warmth", "fuzziness" and "tinglyness". I told her those were feelings associated with relaxation and that this was a good thing!

– Psychologist

I have depression and anxiety attacks. They usually last for a few minutes to a couple of days. They are very intense and at those times I tend to be very depressed and worried. I self-harm at those times and have attempted suicide on more than one occasion.

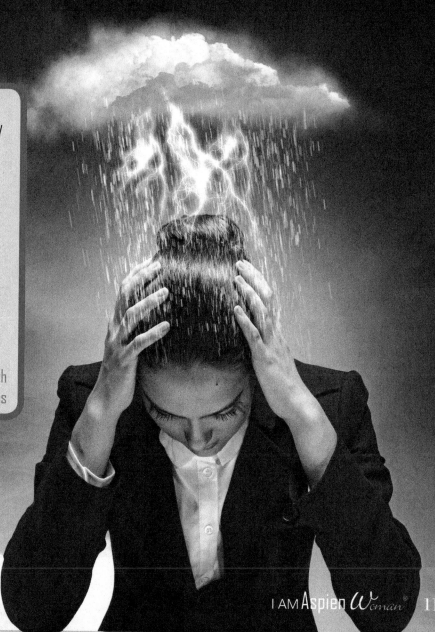

The cause of depression in people on the spectrum can be different to that of typically developing people. Some relevant reasons may be due to being misunderstood, not having the appropriate diagnosis(es), an inability to communicate, invalidation related to the challenges of living with an 'invisible disability' or the diagnostic label, being outcast or bullied by others, lack of self-esteem, self-image and identity, inability to manage change, manage one's emotions, sensory issues and/or finding appropriate and affordable help and support.

– Psychiatrist working with individuals with Autism Spectrum Conditions

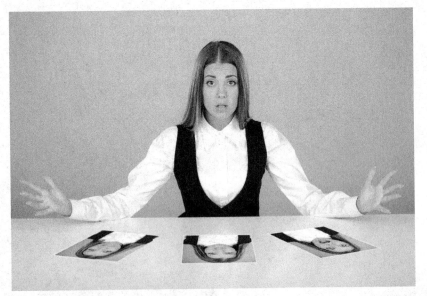

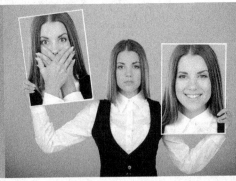

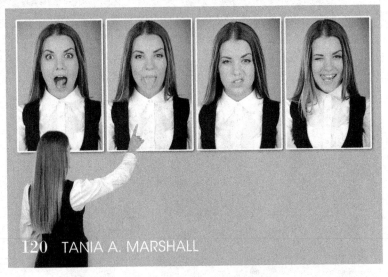

I have alexythymia meaning that I struggle with identifying and describing my emotions.

She has taught herself by taking courses and reading books about emotions, studying faces, emotional intelligence, even micro expressions, how to identify her emotions and feelings and communicate them to others. She is far more emotionally intelligent now than she used to be. It has improved her communications and relationships with others in her career and here at home.
– Partner of emotionally intelligent AspienWoman

Communication/ Language

When it comes to people, I'm usually at my best one-on-one or presenting to others. It wasn't always like that though. I had a lot of anxiety around being looked at and performing in front of others. Working with a therapist really helped me improve.

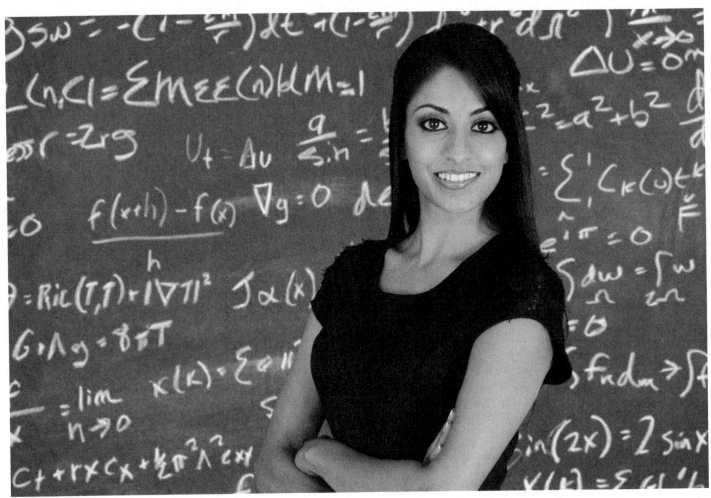

They said she couldn't possibly have Asperger's because she makes good eye contact, can carry on a conversation and has a job. She has learnt and practised eye contact, social skills, nonverbal body language and practised public speaking over and over and over and over ... till it's become a habit. Yes, she has a job but she still makes all sorts of faux pas and still lives at home with us.

– Mother struggling to get a diagnosis for her daughter

I don't do group work. I'm not so good communicating within a group. It all just seems to fall apart and I find it challenging to keep up with everyone and say the right thing at the right time.

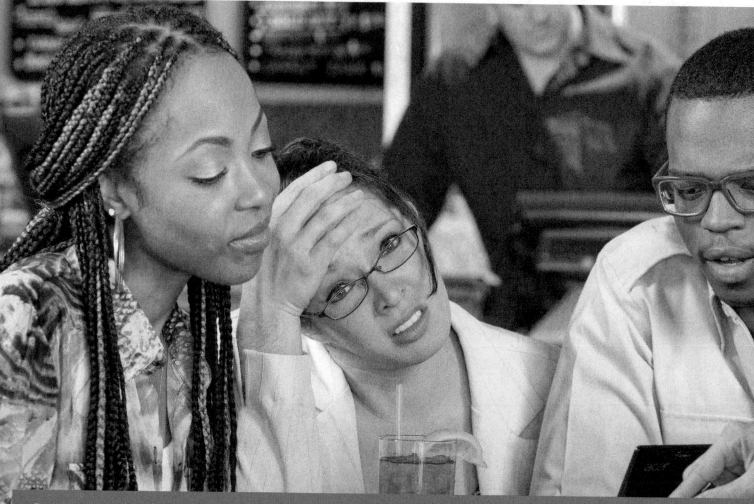

One of her biggest challenges is working with others. Coupled with not understanding the unwritten social rules and the social hierarchy, she has real troubles with being socially appropriate. She recently had an issue with her job and trashed them publicly on Facebook. She got fired, but she still thinks she is right. She has not lasted in a workplace for more than a couple of months.

– Concerned parents of unemployed daughter

When I'm stressed, I tend to shut down and go mute, unable to communicate my feelings and my thoughts in words. I used to have selective mutism when I was a child. I just cannot get the words out. It can still be hard for me today to stop things I don't like by speaking up. I just literally can't think of what to say or do or how to say or do it.

She stresses about little things, big things, future things, past things, things that happened five years ago. She also misinterprets and thinks others are out to get her when they are not. She will often rehash her grievances from a long time ago. I tell her, "But that was five years ago! You need to move on." She is learning to move on and stay in the present through Mindfulness Training.

– Older brother of 19-year-old AspienTeen

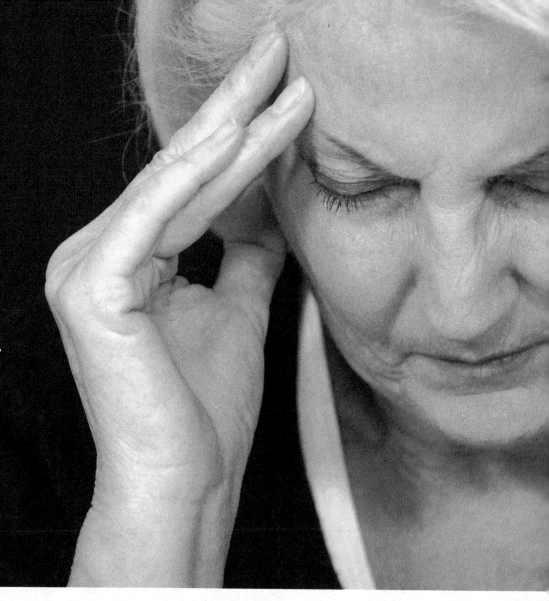

> I rehearse conversations in my mind over and over again. I do this often at night when trying to go to sleep. I play the script, stop, rewind, replay and repeat. I will play back conversations, over and over again, analysing them, to find out where the conversation got derailed or where I might have said the wrong thing. It is exhausting for me.

She really wants to know where the conversation or the interaction went wrong and she just has to find out. At times, she does not get hints, sarcasm or jokes. She has trouble with non-verbal body language and this is why she struggles with relationships and social interactions. At times, she automatically assumes something is about her when maybe it's not. One of her biggest challenges has been her social naivety: believing what people tell her, from world events to the local town gossip. Here she is, this intelligent and brilliant professional artist, who is also highly experienced at jumping to conclusions and making mountains out of molehills.

– Partner of professional artist

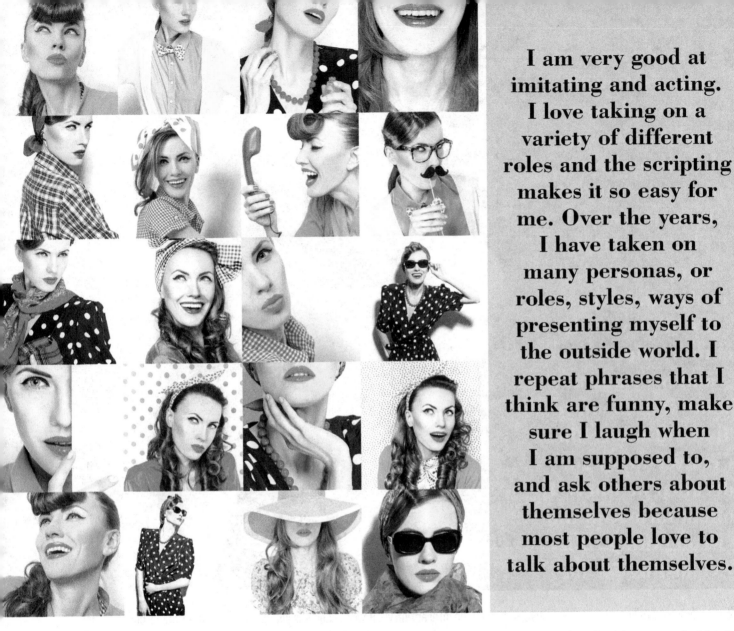

I am very good at imitating and acting. I love taking on a variety of different roles and the scripting makes it so easy for me. Over the years, I have taken on many personas, or roles, styles, ways of presenting myself to the outside world. I repeat phrases that I think are funny, make sure I laugh when I am supposed to, and ask others about themselves because most people love to talk about themselves.

There are a number of compensatory, coping, mimicking, masking, behavioural, verbal and non-verbal body language strategies and scripting that over time many women have used and it is these strategies that can often delay a diagnosis or even prevent a female from receiving the appropriate diagnosis.
— Female Autism researcher

I feel so blessed to be alive today because technology has helped me to be able to communicate better. Before that, it was challenging for me to communicate using words. I text or use social media to my family members and my parents are so much happier that I can communicate better and faster too! At times, I still have trouble verbalising my feelings and asking for help, but it is improving.

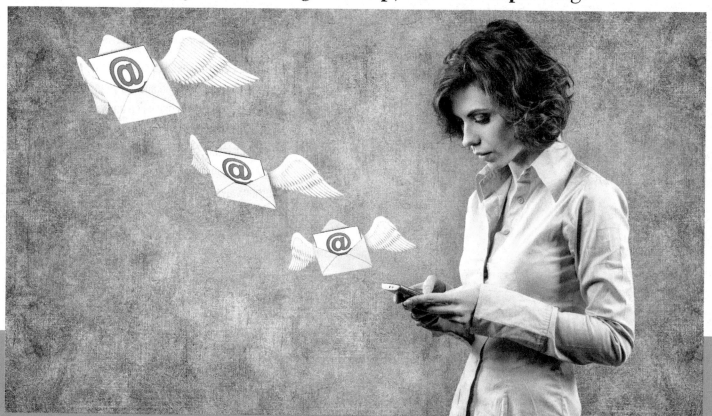

She can write or type her feelings far better than verbalising them. She is great at communicating her innermost experiences using technology. At times, she has appeared to others as 'snobby', 'self-centred' and even 'narcissistic'. She is often misunderstood and has recently discovered that writing is her strength. Speaking ... not so much. We communicate more by writing letters, via text or email. She just entered some of her poetry into a competition. I hope she wins!

– Daughter of mother with newly discovered talent for writing

They say I'm so mature and then they say I'm so immature, I'm such a child? It's so confusing ... why can't they make up their minds? I do dress younger and sound younger than my age. When the phone rings, I often get asked if my mother is there! What's wrong with them?! I really dislike the phone. I have trouble knowing when to talk or not talk. Texting is awesome!

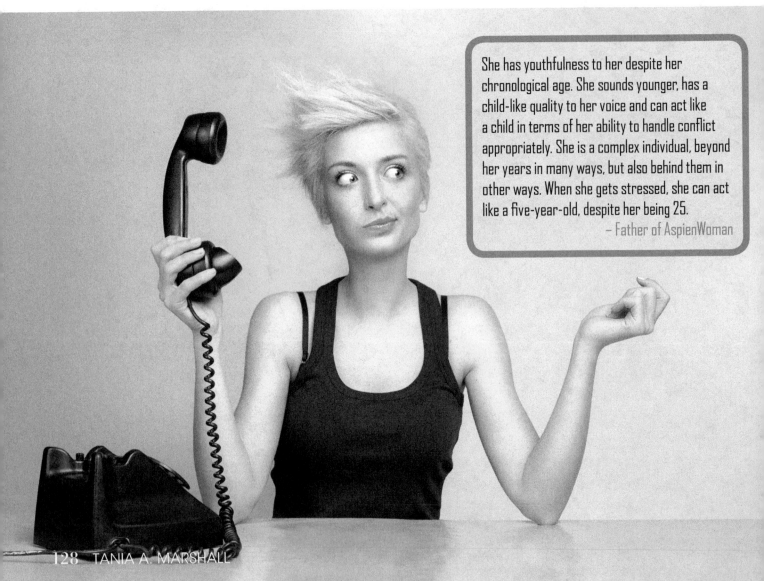

She has youthfulness to her despite her chronological age. She sounds younger, has a child-like quality to her voice and can act like a child in terms of her ability to handle conflict appropriately. She is a complex individual, beyond her years in many ways, but also behind them in other ways. When she gets stressed, she can act like a five-year-old, despite her being 25.
– Father of AspienWoman

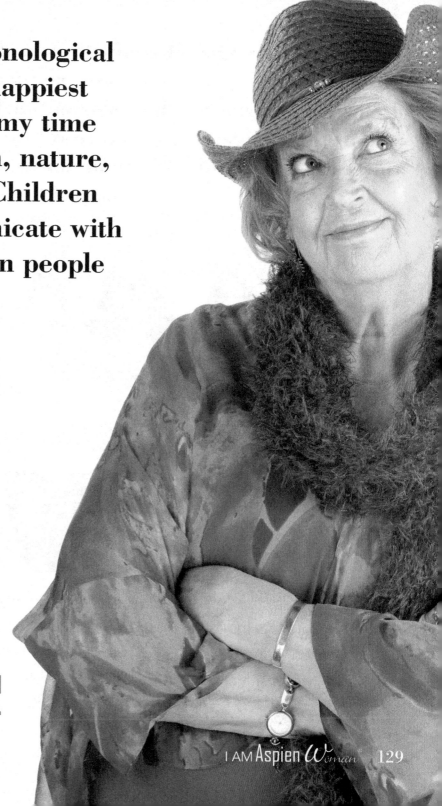

I've never felt my chronological age. I am my most happiest when I am spending my time with animals, children, nature, painting or writing. Children love me! I can communicate with them much better than people my own age.

Grandma is 66 but she doesn't act like it. Just last week she borrowed a brand new shirt of mine to go out somewhere. At family gatherings she's always with the kids and animals. There are a couple of cringeworthy memories I could talk about. Even Mum is embarrassed by her sometimes, but most of the time we think she is so cool.

– 15-year-old granddaughter of talented artistic grandmother

I dislike any kind of conflict intensely and will either avoid it completely or be too aggressive, neither strategy working for me. I used to burn bridges until I started working on myself and learning how to manage, repair and resolve conflict. I took a couple of university counselling and communication skills classes which really helped too.

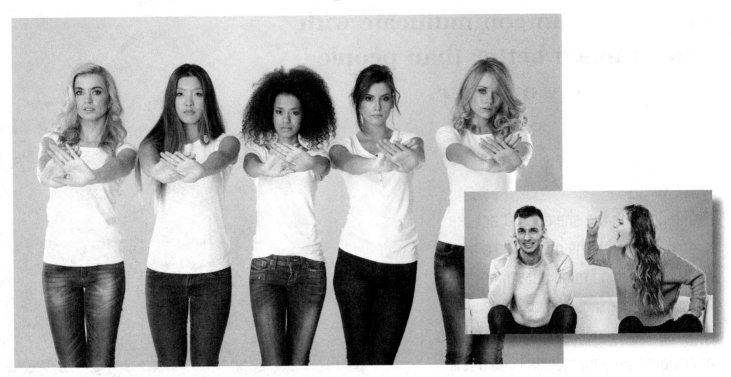

Many women on the spectrum have an inability to resolve conflict, often exploding, blowing things out of proportion, burning bridges and losing friends, jobs and relationships. There is a real need for more professionals to assist them with skills training in distress tolerance, conflict resolution, healthy communication, perspective taking and rigidity of thinking. Many have Borderline Personality Disorder Traits and this is often seen in therapy, with family members and also via social media, in terms of dysfunctional social-communication styles and behaviours.

– Family therapist

I have difficulty communicating with people. I tend to see everyone as on the same level and get in trouble often. I have had to work hard at speaking and communicating in particular ways depending on if it's my boss, my spouse, my children, co-workers or friends. I have been reprimanded a few times at work because of this. I just don't feel it is right to treat one person as more special than another?

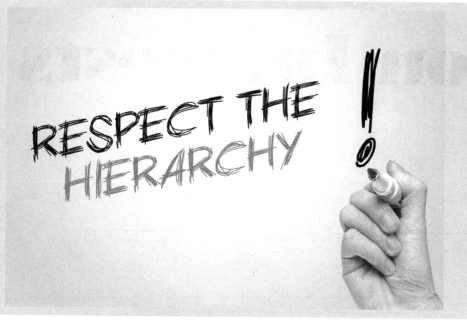

She cannot play the social game. She really is so much more qualified over others but continually gets passed over for promotions due to her inflexibility.

– Partner of self-employed AspienWoman

She recently auditioned for a reality show, but failed to make it through, not because she doesn't have the best voice (in fact, they said she was in the top three), but because she proceeded to tell them what was wrong with their auditioning process! I've tried to explain it to her many times, but it's just not sinking in.

- Mother of Aspie daughter with perfect pitch and gifted voice

Common Interests

I'm a nemophilist. I love the woods, nature, the forest, the solitude, quietness and beauty.

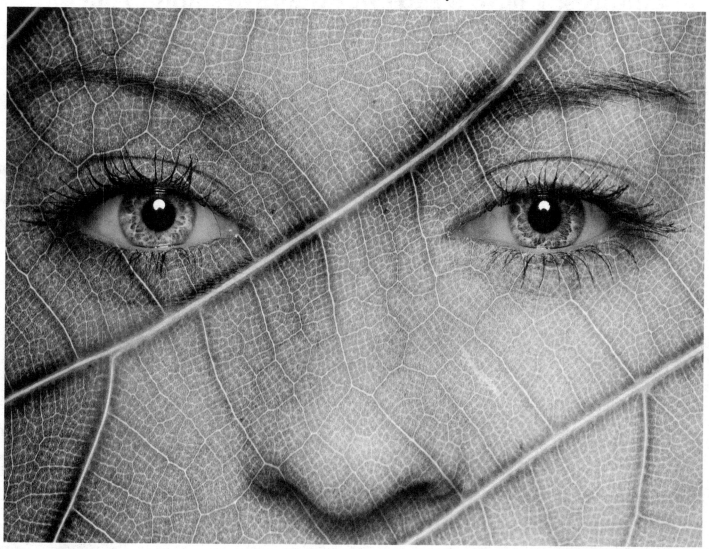

From very early on we saw her passion for nature and animals. She would spend hours out in nature just walking around and studying plants and insects. She is now working in the field of environmental science. It's perfect for her as she has always been concerned about the well-being of the planet.

– Father of 35-year-old

I have always been obsessed with words, languages and cultures. I have a PhD in Linguistics and French.

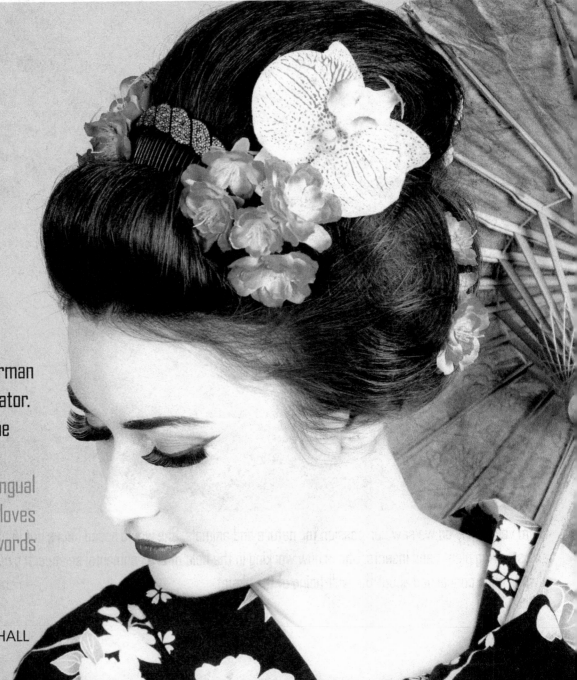

She speaks Spanish, Italian, French and German and works as a translator. She also teaches at the local university.

– Son of multi-lingual mother who loves languages and words

I have travelled all over the world and much further ... with my books. They have taken me to a variety of countries, eras, times, places. I love reading them, smelling them, flicking through the pages. I have an insatiable desire to learn and grow. I read a lot of spiritual, new age and self-help books, paganism and herbalism.

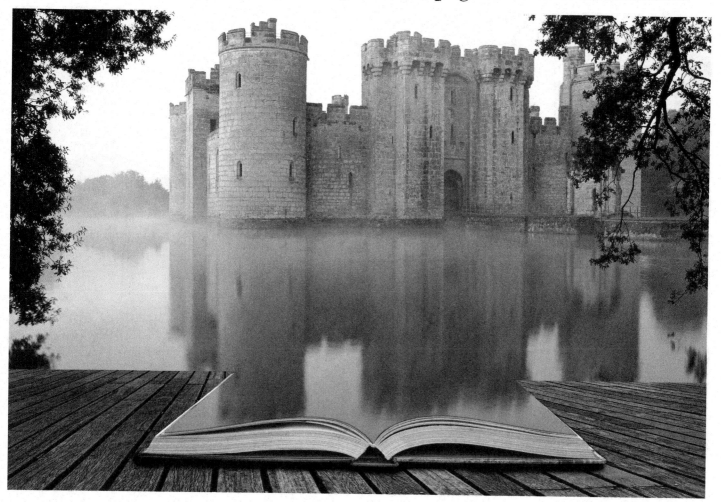

She has always been a bookworm and now she writes them. She just won an award for her best-selling book series. She is a fairly famous author now.

– Niece of best-selling author

I feel as though I am the character at times. I can feel an intense connection with certain characters in books and movies, even falling in love with a character once, but I'd never tell anyone that! I also love writing.

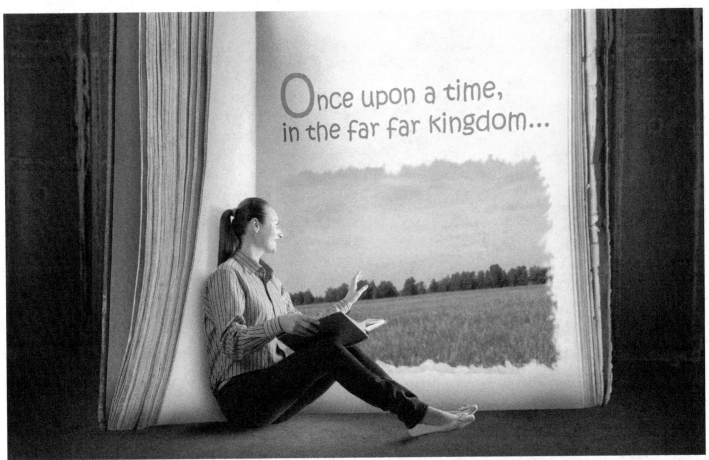

Once upon a time, in the far far kingdom...

She lives inside the book. She loves English literature to the point that her bedroom looks like it came out of Jane Austen's *Pride and Prejudice*. She is in love with the words, the characters, the paper, the pens ... even the smell of the pages.

– Uncle of avid reader

I love technology: working with it, playing games, learning the programming, using it to create something that helps make people's lives better. I have iPhones, iPads, a PC, laptop, iPod, yup ... and a Mac. I love programming, designing websites, anything to do with technology. I just worked on a project where we did the programming for a drone.

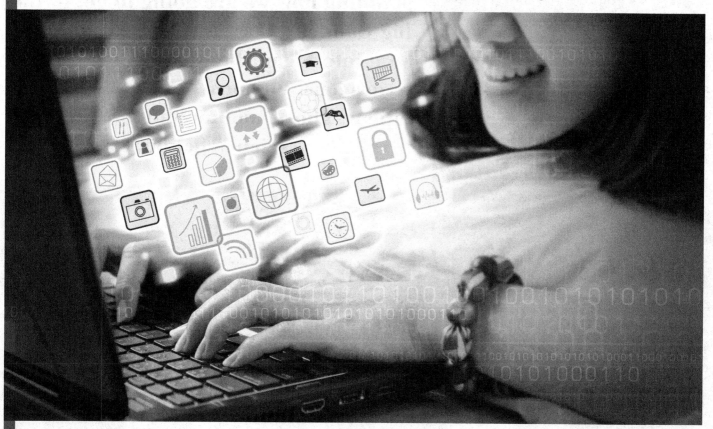

She is a pattern thinker and computer programmer. She says she loves being a part of a team of people that understand her and have similar interests and vice versa. We only hire people with Asperger Syndrome as they are uniquely suited to the positions we have here, which involve programming and solving some pretty big problems at times.

– Director of Technology

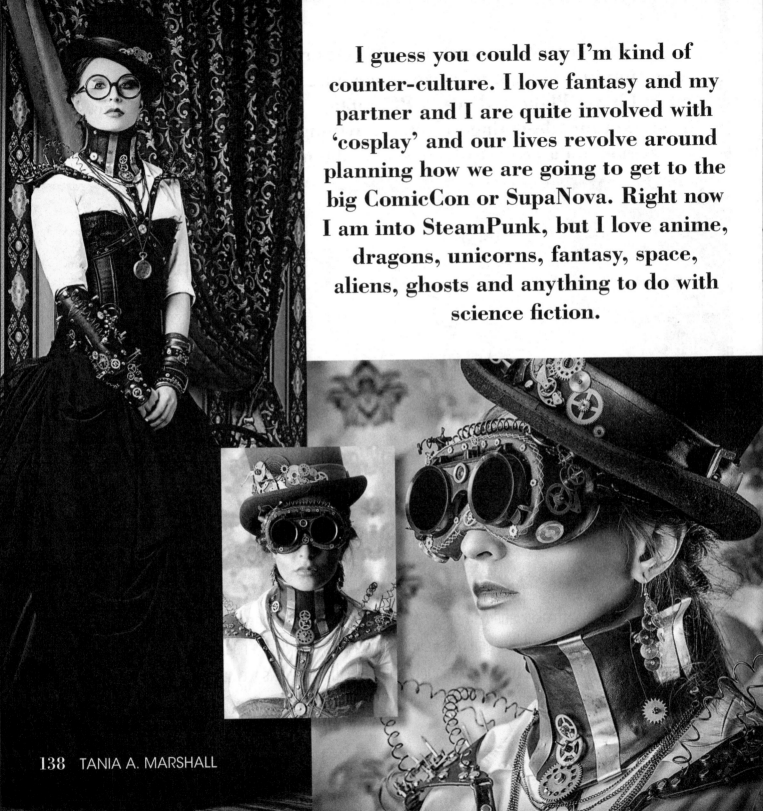

I guess you could say I'm kind of counter-culture. I love fantasy and my partner and I are quite involved with 'cosplay' and our lives revolve around planning how we are going to get to the big ComicCon or SupaNova. Right now I am into SteamPunk, but I love anime, dragons, unicorns, fantasy, space, aliens, ghosts and anything to do with science fiction.

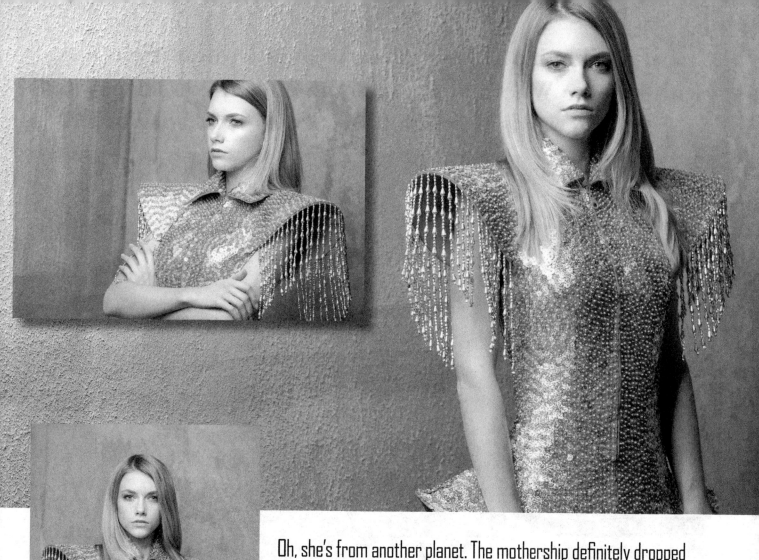

Oh, she's from another planet. The mothership definitely dropped her off here. We all joke about it in our family and she doesn't mind. She's got her own style and people copy it all the time. It drives her crazy. She was always into cosplay and loved to shock my friends with her outfits. She is now a very successful costume designer, so she can get away with dressing like she does ... every day.

– Proud and at times embarrassed conservative brother

I am a Whovian. I have often wished I would time travel with Doctor Who and go on some adventures, backwards and forwards through time. I also love Sherlock.

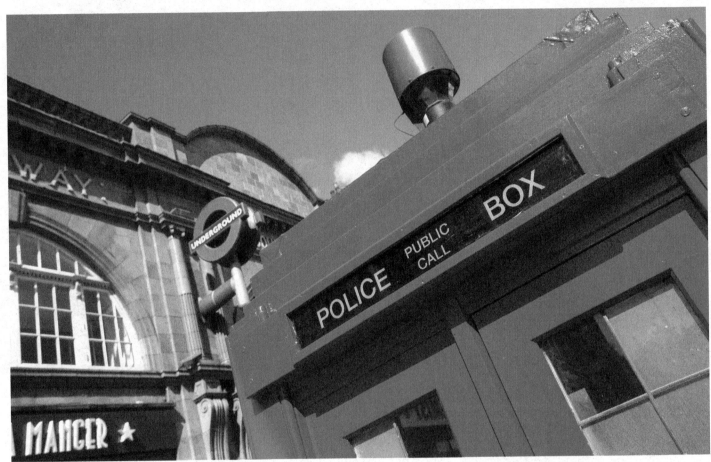

She is a part of an online history group, loves medieval times, *Game of Thrones* stuff, archaeology, linguistics and hieroglyphics. She is particularly interested in Egyptology and now teaches it at university.

– Daughter of archaeologist mother

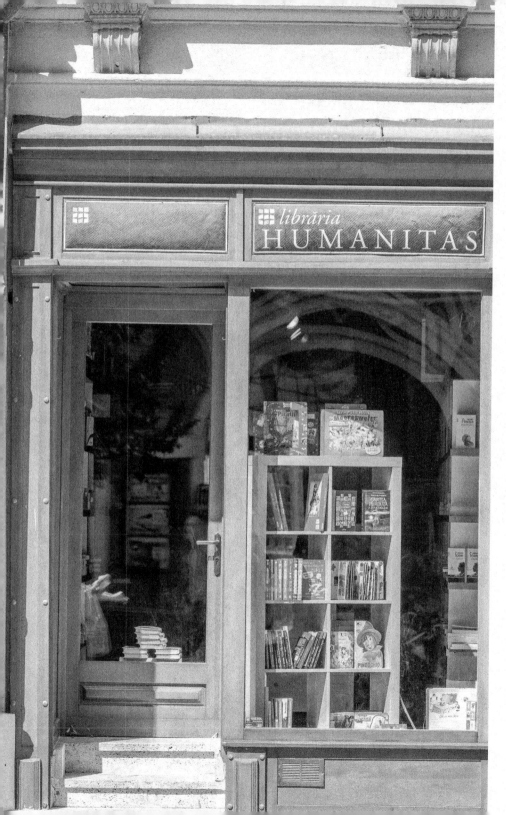

Psychology (and psychiatry), philosophy and education has always been my passion and has been ever since I was really young. I have always been intrigued by human behaviour and what makes people tick. Where do we come from? Why are we here? Where are we going? Why do people do what they do?

From very young she has asked us the BIG questions and we didn't know the answers. So she read and studied and read and studied. She does find it difficult at times because she wants the answers to life in very black-and-white ways. She loves the rules and when things don't make sense, she can get frustrated.

– Stepmother of curious psychology student

I love participating in medieval festivals. There's the dressing up, the acting, the horses and the entertaining. I can't socialise much but I love entertaining others. I go by my scripts and lines and there's nothing else more satisfying for me than performing in front of others.

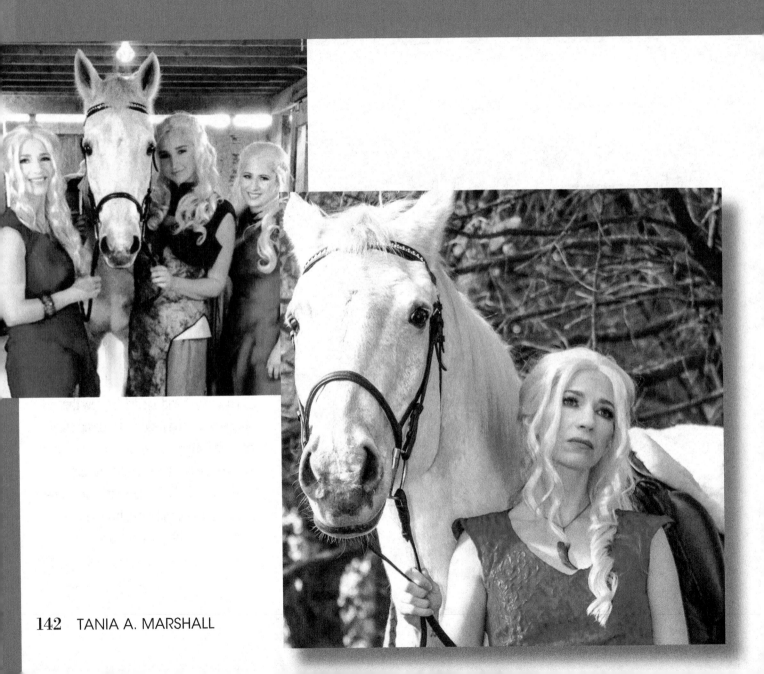

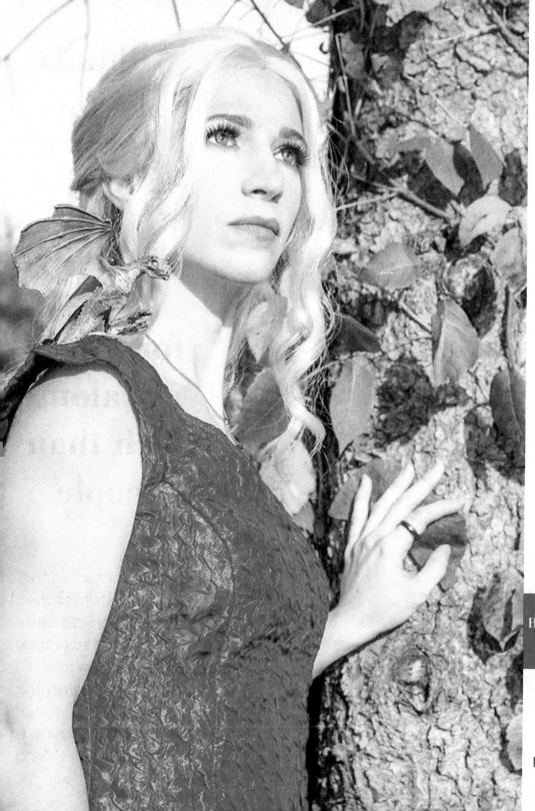

Her love for other worlds started when she was very young. She has always been very interested in other times, other cultures and other eras. She says they are far more interesting than present-day life.

– Mother of daughter living in fantasy worlds

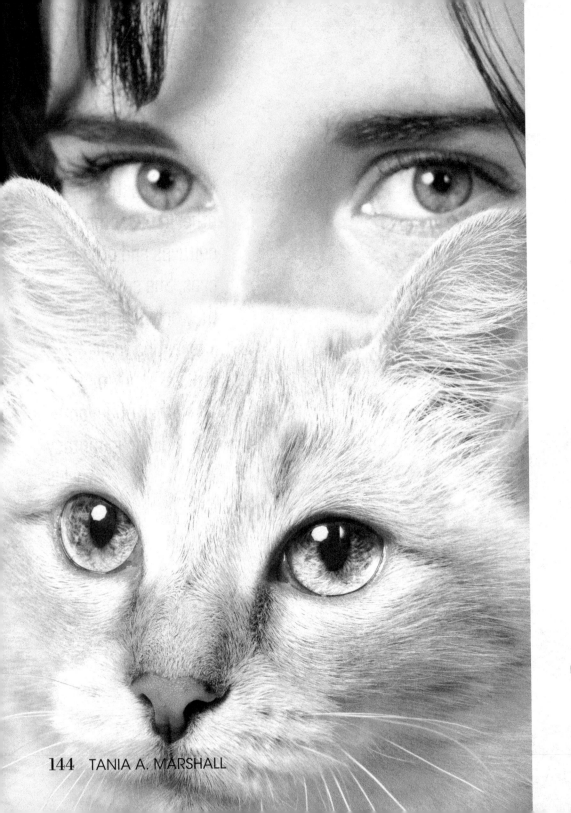

Animals are my best friends and much easier for me to get along with than people.

She is known as the cat lady, rescuing cats from here and there and everywhere. She has now started up a cat adoption centre out of her own home, with a website and everything.
– Best friend to a 50-year-old female with a recent diagnosis of Autism

My pets *are* members of the family

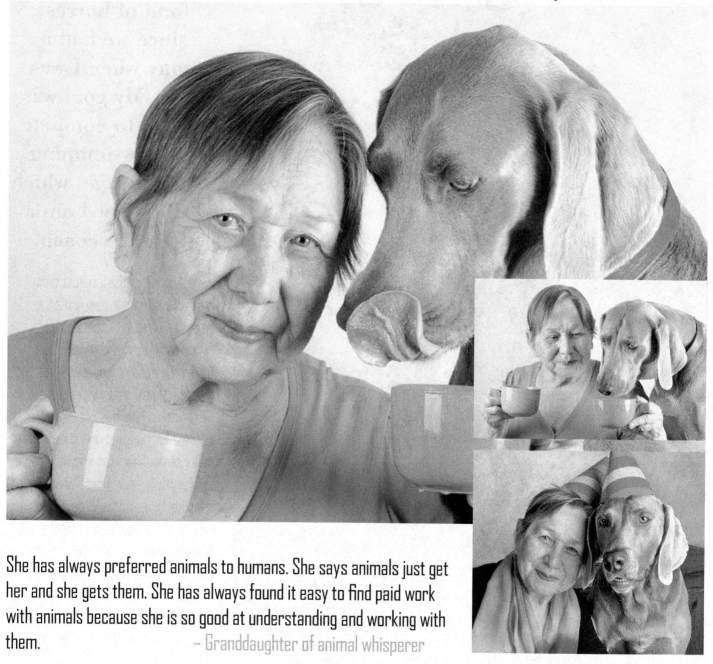

She has always preferred animals to humans. She says animals just get her and she gets them. She has always found it easy to find paid work with animals because she is so good at understanding and working with them.
              – Granddaughter of animal whisperer

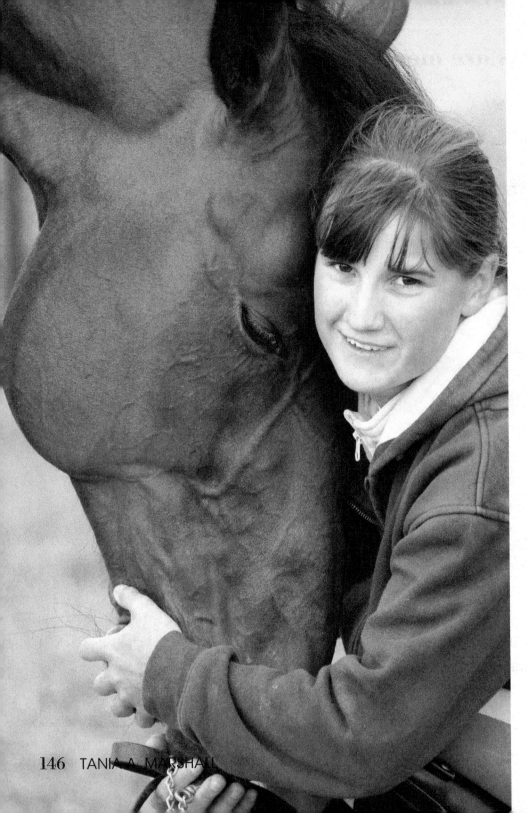

I have always been fond of horses, since we had a pony when I was little. My goal was always to compete in show-jumping and dressage, which I did. Now I am a dressage coach.

It's not so much the interest that is different to their peers, it's the intensity. A recent client brought in her scrapbook and as I leafed through it became apparent that my client knew everything about her interest. She had taken and successfully passed online courses in horsemanship, was knowledgeable in everything from horse anatomy, to training, types and breeds of horses, temperament, different heights, horses' speed, saddlery and much more. She has her own pony and attends pony club. Her goal is to have her own farm and teach others about horses. She is well on her way to her dream.

– Psychologist

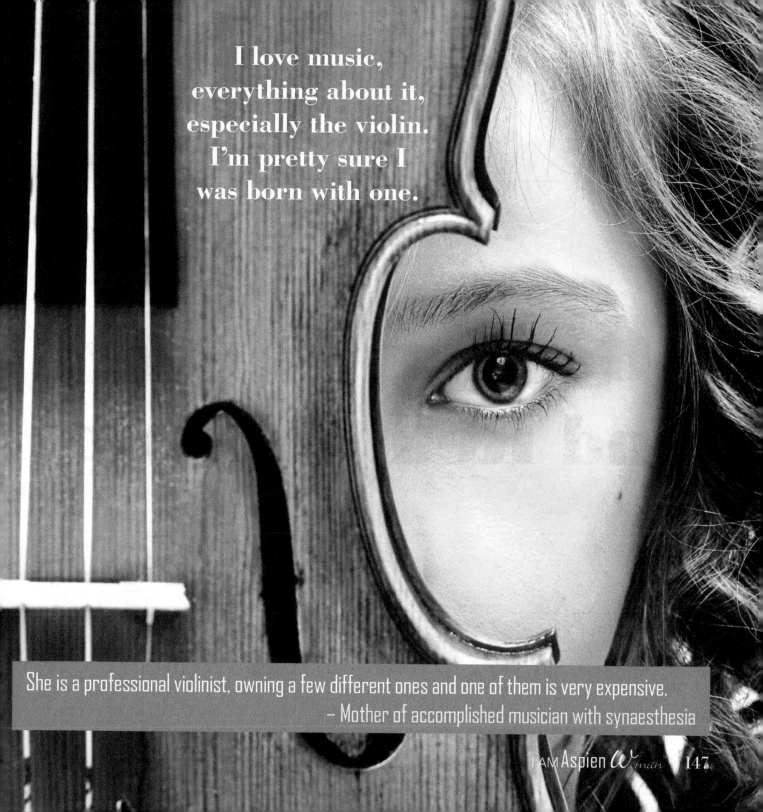

I love music,
everything about it,
especially the violin.
I'm pretty sure I
was born with one.

She is a professional violinist, owning a few different ones and one of them is very expensive.
– Mother of accomplished musician with synaesthesia

Gender, Family and Relationships

We are twins on the spectrum! I have always dressed as a tomboy. At the age of 16, I cut off my hair and told everyone I wanted to be a guy. I had been living online as a guy for a while and found that people seemed to like me. My sister has not had any gender or sexuality issues.

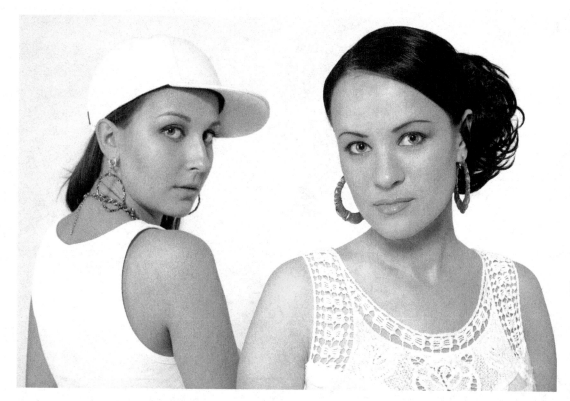

I have not had any gender or sexuality issues although my sister and her friends identify as transgender. They refer to people like me as cisgender, who were both born with female characteristics and identify as a woman or are not transgender.

Individuals with an Autism Spectrum Condition are more likely to experience gender dysphoria/gender identity disorder (GID) and the number of gay lesbian, gay, bisexual, transgender and intersex (LGBTI) are anecdotally higher. Some new research is starting to find these results as well. Sometimes the feeling of 'not fitting in' or feeling 'different' is attributed to the wrong gender rather than it being Autism. For some individuals, it may be having a different experience of gender identity or placing less importance on the social aspects of gender (seeing the person first, and then the gender, age and/or shared interests).

– Autistic researcher (area of Autism)

I am gender-fluid. I don't feel like I identify fully as a female or a male. I didn't know it was possible to me that I could be a 'girl', with all the external evidence pointing against it and all the internal evidence pointing towards it. But I've always known I don't have an ounce of masculinity in me. I just didn't know how to get to womanhood without being killed or benefitting from magic or the technology of an advanced alien civilisation.

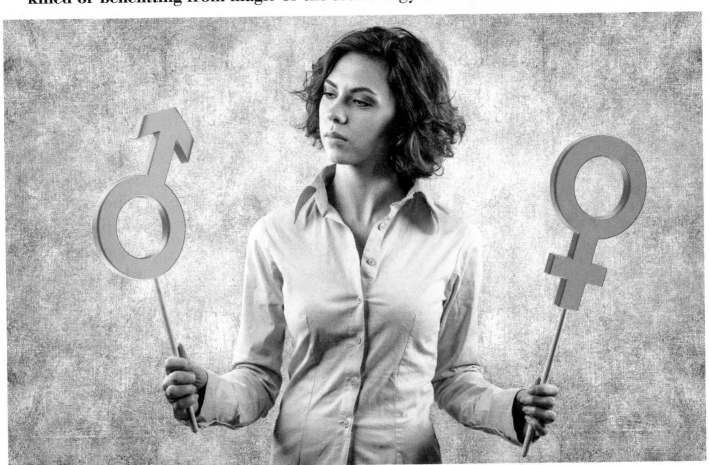

Some individuals feel as though they are gender blind, agender or genderless. Some are born female but have always felt male, some dress similar to males, and some may identify as women but have no interest in 'masculine' and/or 'feminine' behaviours and interests. Some refer to themselves as part of the pansexual or omnisexual population, referring to gender-blindness. This means that they see the person first and gender and sex are not relevant in terms of who they are sexually, romantically or emotionally attracted to.
— Psychiatrist specialising in sexuality and gender

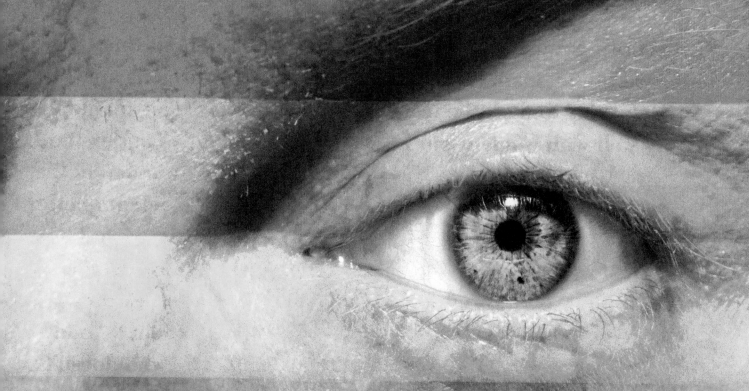

A smaller group of us are LGTB or lesbian, gay, transgender and bisexual. An umbrella term that is used to refer to the community as a whole is LGBTQIA and also includes the queer, intersex and asexual communities under our umbrella.

Approximately 1% of the general population are intersex and are born that way. This means that they were not born with all of the biological characteristics of male or female or they might have a combination of those characteristics. Those who refer to themselves as asexual do not typically experience being sexually attracted to others.

– LGBTQIA advocate

I was born a female, there's certainly no doubt about that, but I am sure I am a man, a gay man, very fashion conscious and I do love clothing and all the trends! Problem is, gay men get along really well with women, but I never have, although I understand women on the spectrum better. So, here I am: I'm a gay man stuck inside a female body who doesn't get along with females and I feel very confused by it all.

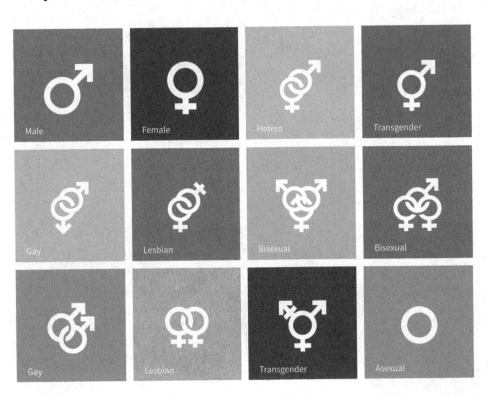

Women who are transgender or gender diverse are more likely to be homeless or at risk of homelessness and this is a big concern for us. Our gender centre offers a range of services for transgender and gender diverse people, their families, their partners and friends.

– Director, gender identity specialist clinic

I grew up with gender identity issues: girl on the outside and boy on the inside. The feelings that came with my confusion were painful and I kept it secret for many years. I am not transgender, but was desperately seeking acceptance in any form I could. Now I still do consider myself to have many androgynous traits and have never been a stereotypical female. But I am for the most part happy with the body I am in and no longer wish to be the opposite sex. It's been a lifetime of struggle for me. I still feel like a man in a dress when I try to fit in with other women.

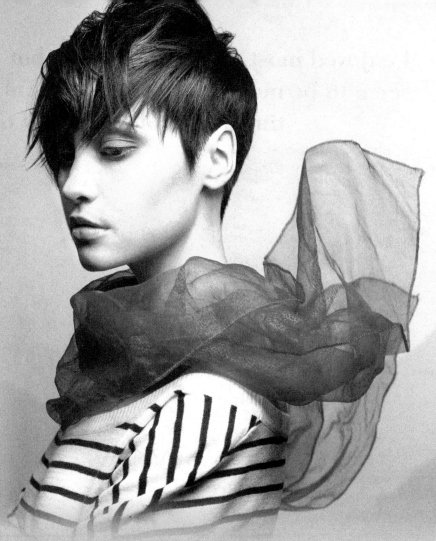

Back then we were as confused as she was. This is an issue that needs to be addressed and people with similar challenges are in desperate need of assistance, support and care, especially in the areas of acceptance and understanding and embracing their identity. She is in a great long-term relationship now, but for a while there I think she believed real life and relationships are like they are in books. We have had many chats because her viewpoint on romantic relationships tends to be more idealistic and based on books.

– Mother of agender 30-year-old writer and author

I enjoyed most of my pregnancy, but my sensory issues did seem to be more apparent to me and to others during that time of my life than any other time.

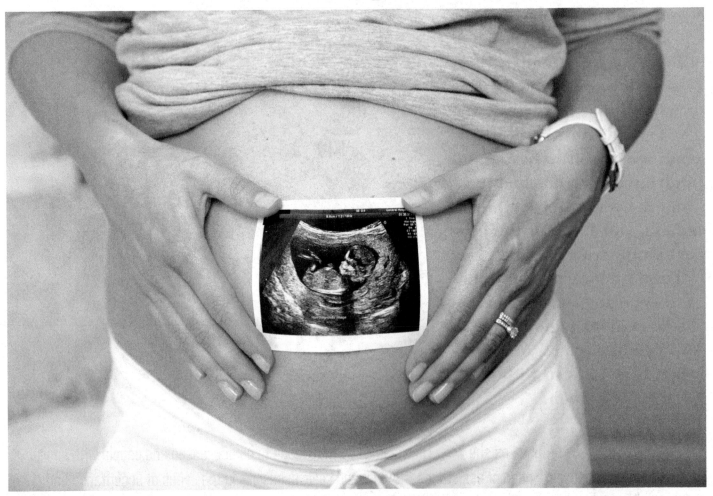

She is sensitive to crying and screaming and does get overwhelmed at times, but she is a great mother and has learnt some techniques that assist her. She wears ear plugs and the kids try hard to be a bit quieter. She now finds it less challenging to meet our children's needs when they are screaming.

– Partner of AspienWoman mother

I love being a mother and I found the experience of it mostly positive. They made all kinds of allowances and modifications in the birthing room, which made all the difference for me. I do know some other mothers on the spectrum who really struggle with motherhood. One in particular has great difficulty sensory processing-wise. Her children are all over her much of the time and she says she needs her space.

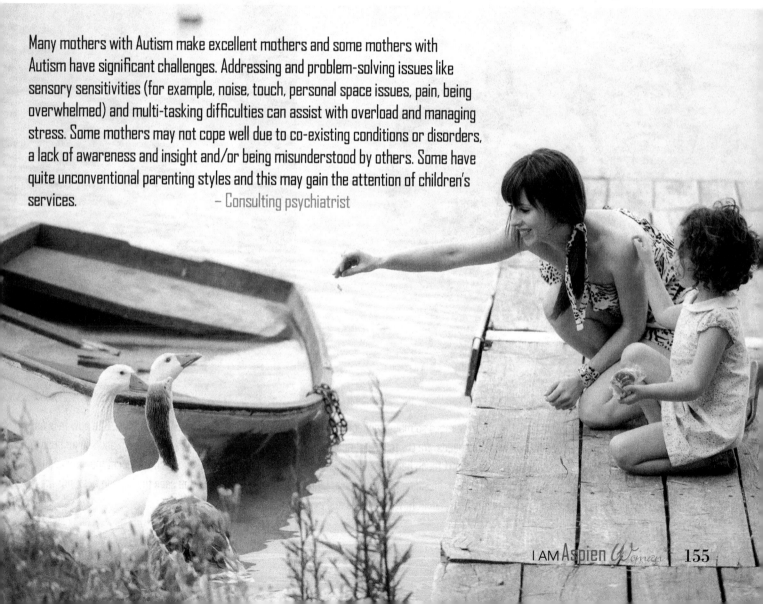

Many mothers with Autism make excellent mothers and some mothers with Autism have significant challenges. Addressing and problem-solving issues like sensory sensitivities (for example, noise, touch, personal space issues, pain, being overwhelmed) and multi-tasking difficulties can assist with overload and managing stress. Some mothers may not cope well due to co-existing conditions or disorders, a lack of awareness and insight and/or being misunderstood by others. Some have quite unconventional parenting styles and this may gain the attention of children's services. — Consulting psychiatrist

I am 58 and cannot understand anyone my age. I think my traits have gotten more profound and obvious as I get older. My stimming (self-soothing) is worse and pretending to be normal is more challenging. What becomes of people over 40 with Asperger's and then into the 50s and 60s? I feel like as I get older, the expectations to 'be normal' and 'fit in' is also higher. Some Aspies may 'grow out' of things or learn to function better but my Asperger troubles seem to be growing worse, as I now have health problems.

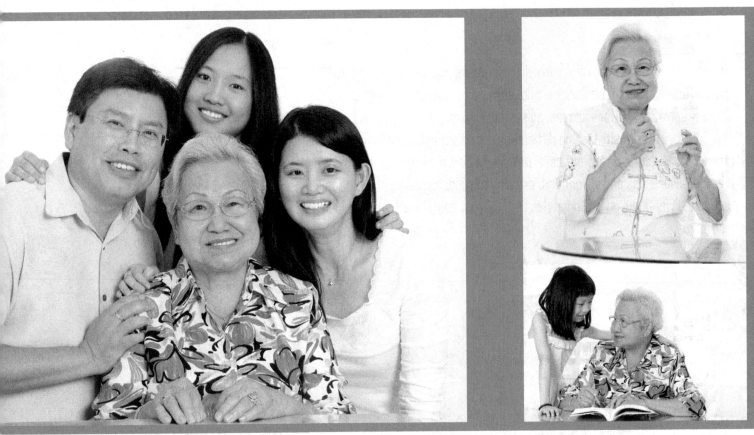

The more we read and understand Autism, the more we make so many connections; this has brought us understanding and peace. She now tells us when she is sensory overloaded and tells us what she needs. We try to keep it peaceful, but the kids always want to sit on her lap and she just can't do that. She says she hates having to tell them that they can't touch her. She also thinks about love as 'boundary-less', which we learnt means the ability to love people of any age, religion, appearance and gender, including gender-mobile (androgynous, transsexual). She sees the person first, not the age, for example. The diagnosis has explained so much to us all about how she thinks and experiences the world.

– Adult daughter of newly diagnosed grandmother

I struggle having to socialise with all the other mums. I do it for the children, but it really does challenge me.

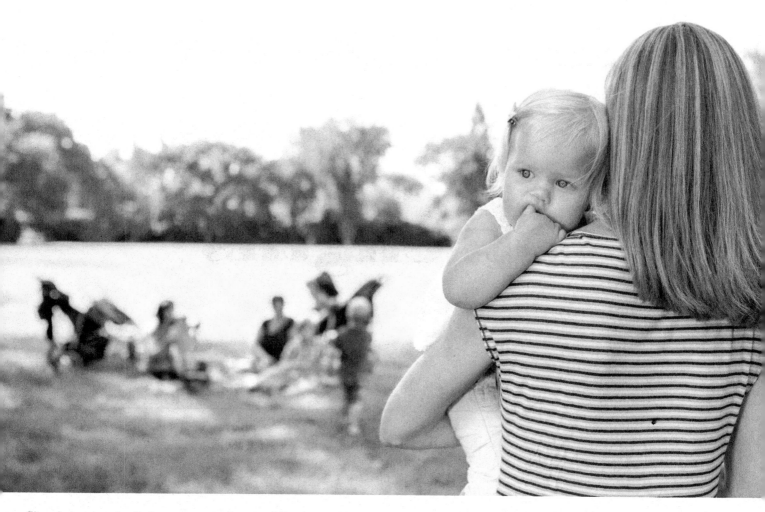

She often says she feels pressure to be social for our children's sake and because she doesn't want them to have the same experiences as her, but she was only recently diagnosed and the children were diagnosed much younger than she was. She often feels so confused that she ends up either not saying anything or talking too much, usually about the things she's passionate about, but unfortunately her peers just don't understand her lifelong struggles and she doesn't know how to tell them.

– Partner of AspienMum

Strengths

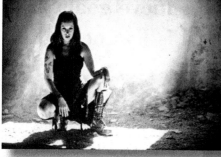

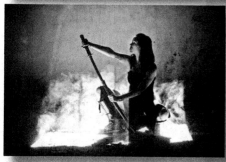

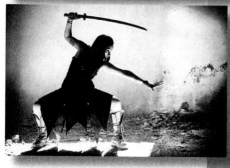

I had my first depression as a child, was institutionalised as a teenager for a while, went to university and finally finished my fourth degree, had another breakdown and suicide attempt, lost jobs, friends and money. I've overcome drug and alcohol addiction, come clean, and now work with people with Autism, just like me. They tell me all the time how resilient I am. I'm surprised I'm still alive.

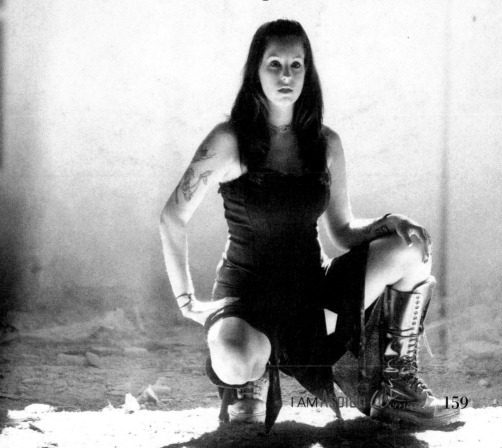

Many adults with Autism are undiagnosed, struggling day to day, yet display an amazing resilience to life's challenges, despite having been through a number of depressive episodes, work and/or social or personal failures. There is a higher rate of suicidal ideation/ suicide in individuals with an Autism Spectrum Condition.

– Director,
Autism spectrum psychology centre

I would describe myself as pretty determined. I achieve goals with intent and purpose, once I've figured out what it is I want to do.

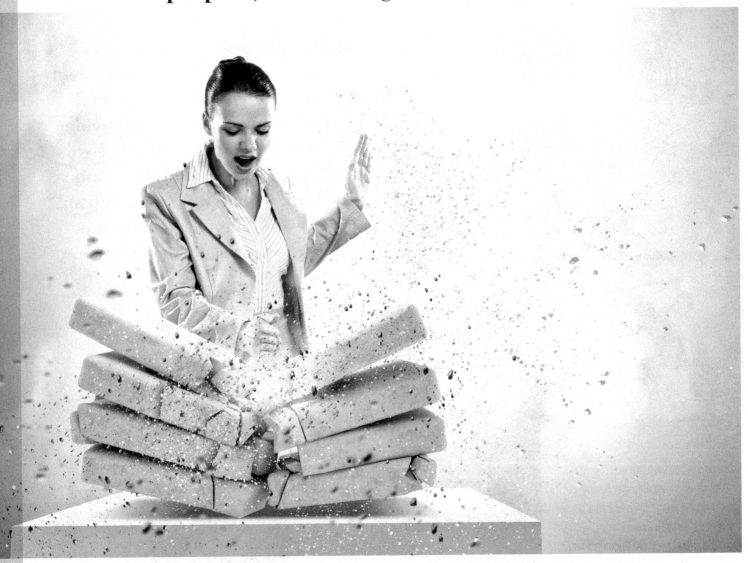

Go hard or go home is her motto. Once she sets her mind on a goal, you can be guaranteed she will achieve it. It's amazing watching her achievements over time. She is a successful entrepreneur.

– Parents of self-employed daughter

I love learning and teaching myself how to do things. I am a self-taught programmer, both Spanish and Italian and dance choreography and have an Intelligence Quotient of 151. I don't like others teaching me because I like to do it myself and my own way. I have also taught myself to make all kinds of craft and I make my own scarfs.

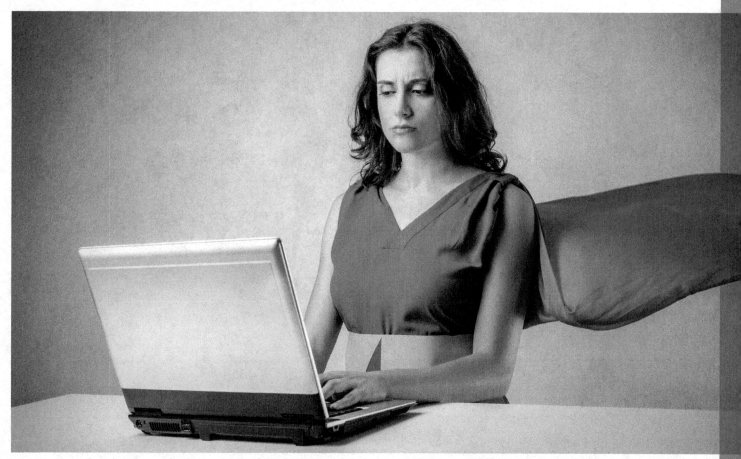

We remember when she started school and she wouldn't let the teacher teach her. At the time we couldn't understand why, but over time we learnt that she works best when given the work with some scaffolding. As a child she was always playing the role of a teacher, never the student.

– Parents of strong-willed adult daughter

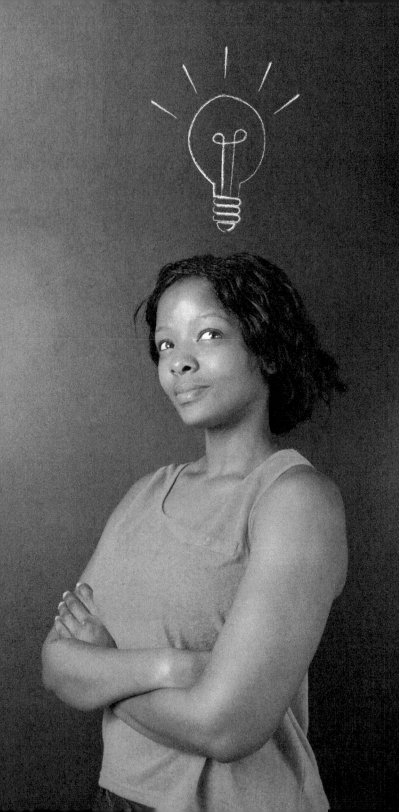

I think outside the box. I can come up with all kinds of creative solutions. I don't know where they come from, but they just come into my head and out my mouth. I've always had lots of ideas. They call me an idea generator.

She is always coming up with ideas for what to do, create, invent and has made some of them come into fruition. She's a smart cookie, that one.
— Self-taught engineer and grandfather

I am a best-selling author. I can sit and write for days, often without showering or having a break. It is called hyperfocus.

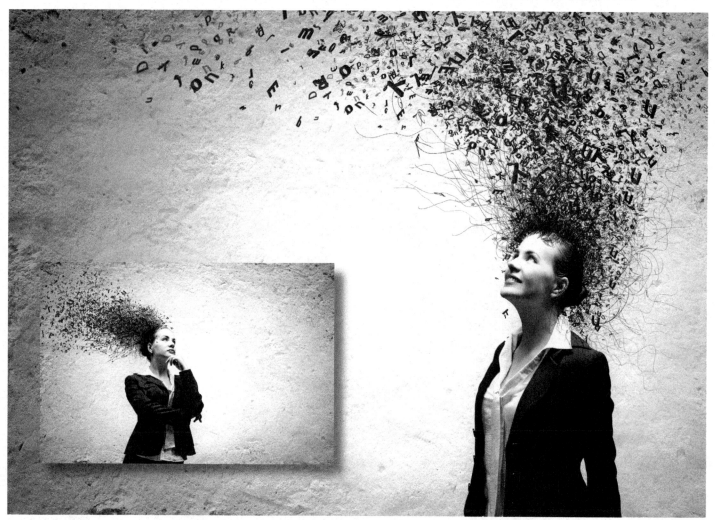

I've known many an individual on the spectrum to hyperfocus on their interest for hours or days at a time, often completing anything from a huge jigsaw puzzle to a drawing to an entire book. It is truly incredible to see them create like that, an entire book or painting in that short of a period.

– Educational psychologist

I love to make people laugh, but I'm not so good when they laugh at me. They say they are laughing with me. I like my sense of humour.

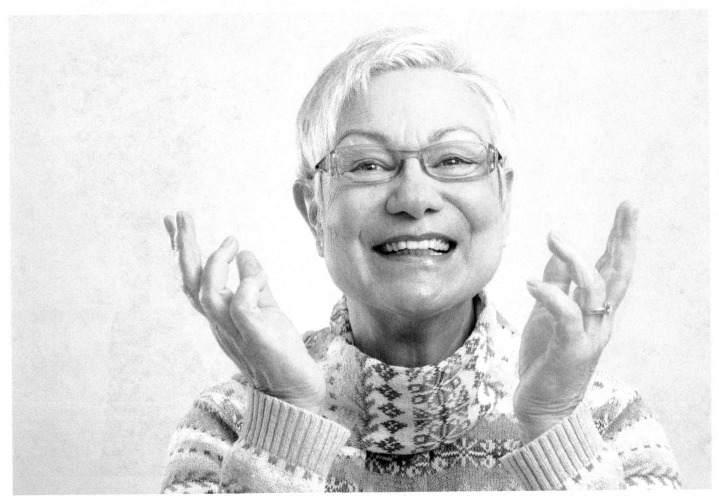

She has a great sense of humour. She can come up with the most amazing comebacks and responses ... two days later ... it's frustrating for her but she can have us all in stitches.

– Family of comedian and self-diagnosed grandmother

I am a professional photographer and photo editor. My intense focus on how the light falls, the lines and attention to detail give my pictures soul and life.

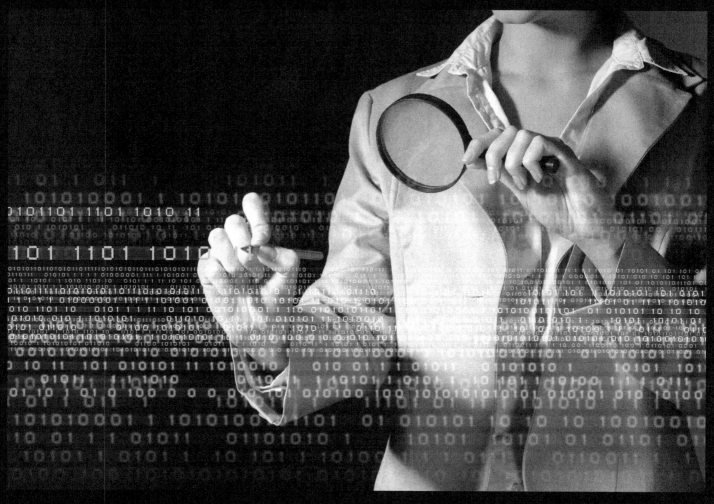

She has always been able to 'see' what others don't see. When you look at her pictures you can see what she focuses on, whether it's the lines or the raindrops or the way the light falls, as she describes it. She has won some photography competitions.

— Twin daughters of professional photographer

I am a hardworking, persistent perfectionistic and put in 110%. I have always been that way and I just can't seem to help it. I'm learning some boundaries now because my children have told me I work too much.

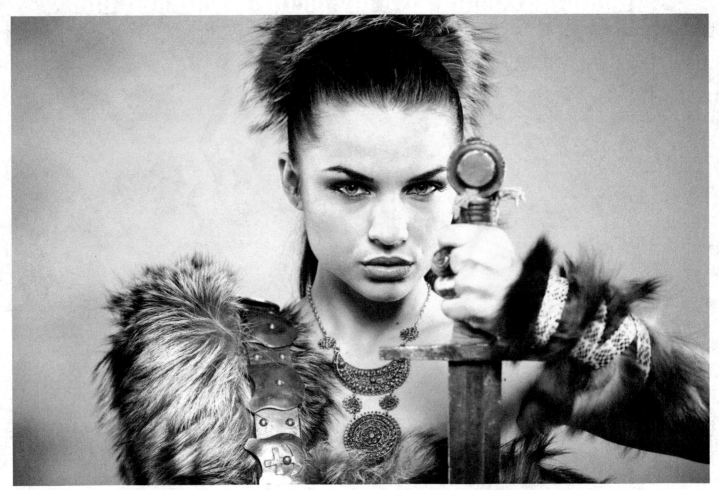

When she has set her mind on something she will achieve her goal. She knows she works harder than her co-workers but she says she can't help it, she likes to do a great job at everything she does. It used to frustrate her but now she understands that some people just work to do their job and then go home. She's better at research than the CIA!

– Children of hardworking AspienWoman

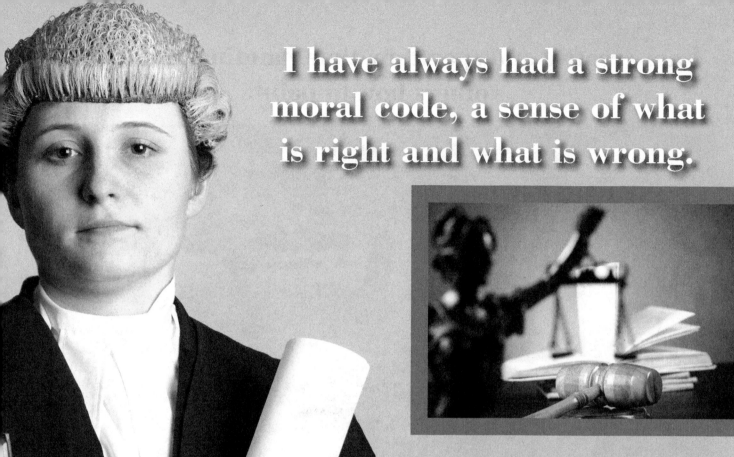

I have always had a strong moral code, a sense of what is right and what is wrong.

She means what she says, does what she says and is honest. She wants the world to be better and she doesn't accept anything less than 100%. She lives her values and wants everything she does to be right and meaningful.

— Partner of AspienWoman lawyer

I am creative and spend my time painting and teaching others how to paint.

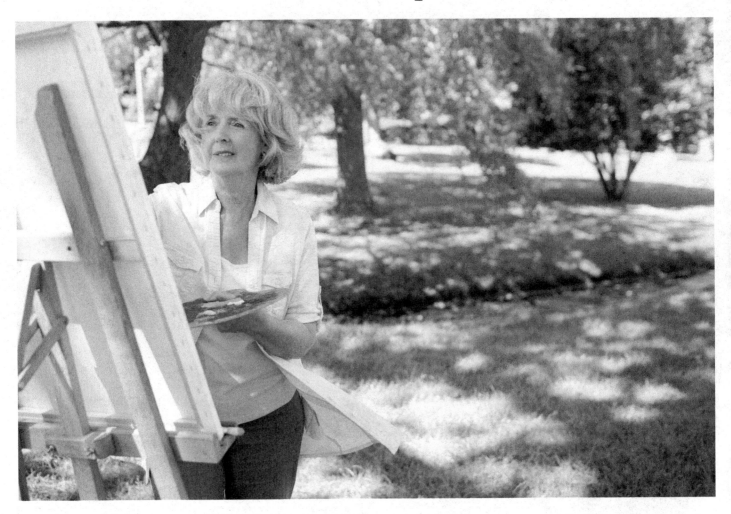

She has ideas no one else has thought of. She wakes up from a dream and has an idea to start an art project or devise a new system. She sees things differently than others. She can take photographs, design, sing, draw, paint and write. She has made her own clothing and made her own skin products from natural ingredients. She never does things the usual way. She is also a born entrepreneur.

– Mother of late-diagnosed artist

I love to research things I am interested in. This has helped to become an expert in the field of medicine.

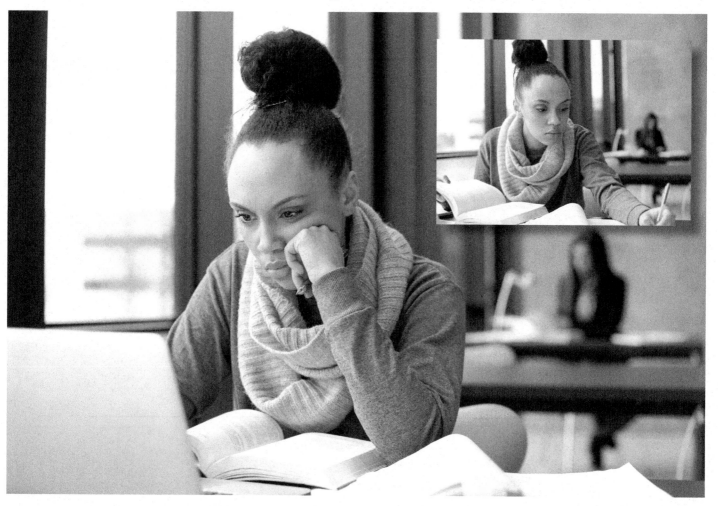

She has always been able to focus for very long periods of time on one thing, collecting knowledge and information, organising and planning. She's always doing research on the computer and mobile phone, reading or writing. She eventually becomes an expert and then moves on to the next subject she's interested in.

– Teen son of self-diagnosed professor

Challenges

It has always been exhaustive to be so good, with the effort to be obedient and try to be so well behaved all the time. It never occurred to me to not follow the rules and I am learning that just because something comes from an authority figure doesn't mean it's safe. I am socially naive and tend to believe things that people tell me and what I hear about people from others.

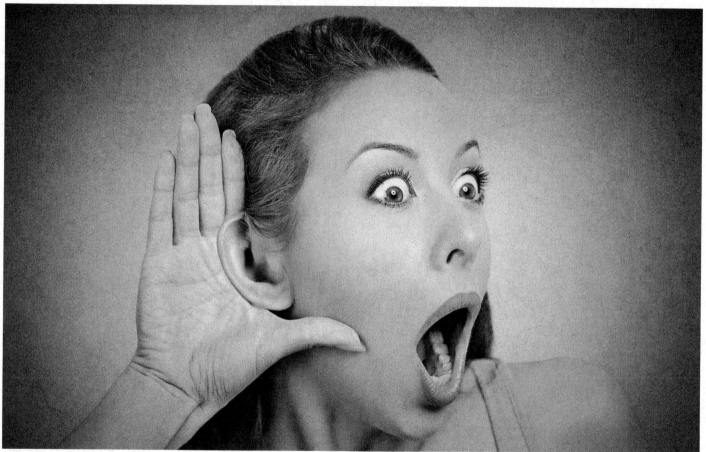

When we were kids, we used to play all kinds of jokes on her. She was ... no, still she is ... so gullible. We would make up all kinds of stories about people at school and she'd believe us. One time though, our tricks backfired and she got in big trouble because of us, but back then we had no idea she'd take us so seriously. I mean our stories were ... we thought they were so obviously made up. We all joke about it now, but my brother and I still feel bad about it.

– Mischievous brothers of naive AspienSister

I struggle with stress, emotions, overwhelm, overload and overthinking. I was on the path to self-destruction. Overthinking and having my mind on the negative or the past is something I am working on. Many times I have hated the fact that I seem to need answers to every daft brainwave I have. Life would be easier if all I cared about was the latest handbag!

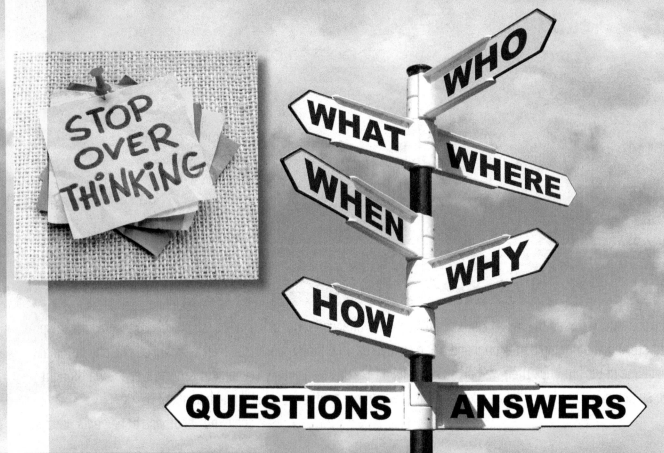

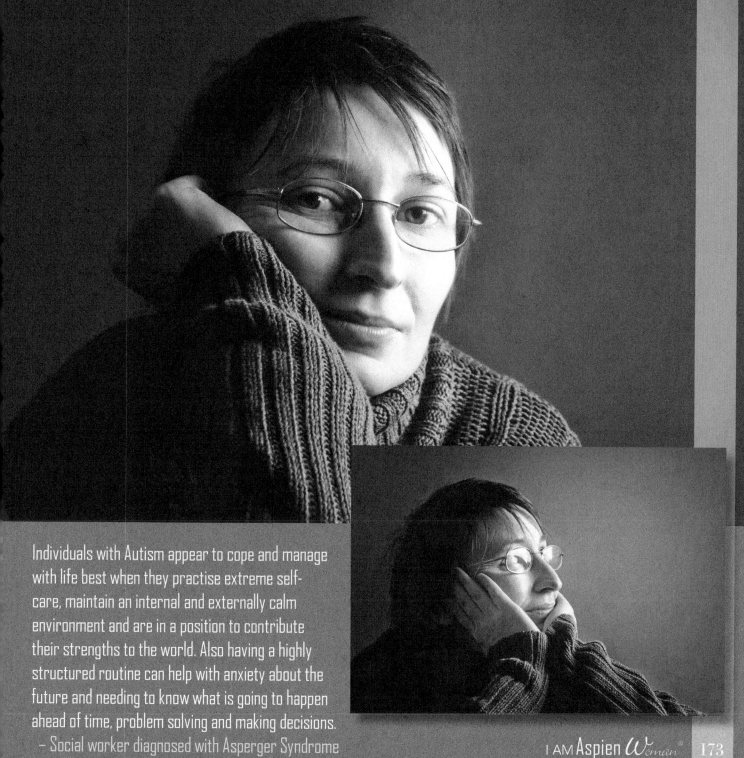

Individuals with Autism appear to cope and manage with life best when they practise extreme self-care, maintain an internal and externally calm environment and are in a position to contribute their strengths to the world. Also having a highly structured routine can help with anxiety about the future and needing to know what is going to happen ahead of time, problem solving and making decisions.

– Social worker diagnosed with Asperger Syndrome

My life hasn't been an easy one. It took me until age 40 when I felt like I had it all figured out and actually started enjoying life. That was after my formal diagnosis and receiving assistance and support. My biggest issue is managing stress and anxiety.

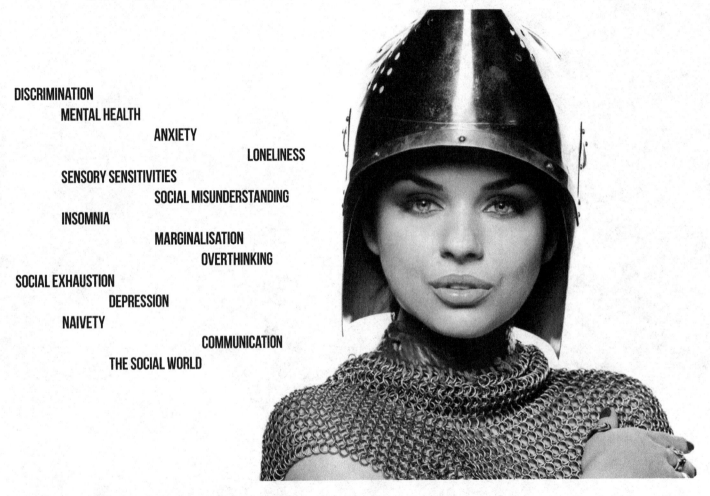

DISCRIMINATION
MENTAL HEALTH
ANXIETY
LONELINESS
SENSORY SENSITIVITIES
SOCIAL MISUNDERSTANDING
INSOMNIA
MARGINALISATION
OVERTHINKING
SOCIAL EXHAUSTION
DEPRESSION
NAIVETY
COMMUNICATION
THE SOCIAL WORLD

Many females are twice marginalised. Being female with a different way of seeing the world can be a very lonely place to be. A formal diagnosis and support can change and save lives.

– Psychiatrist

I've always found it hard to understand people. They don't say what they mean or mean what they say, spend too much time chit-chatting and some people are just plain stupid! I am learning to be less rigid and negative and more flexible in my thinking.

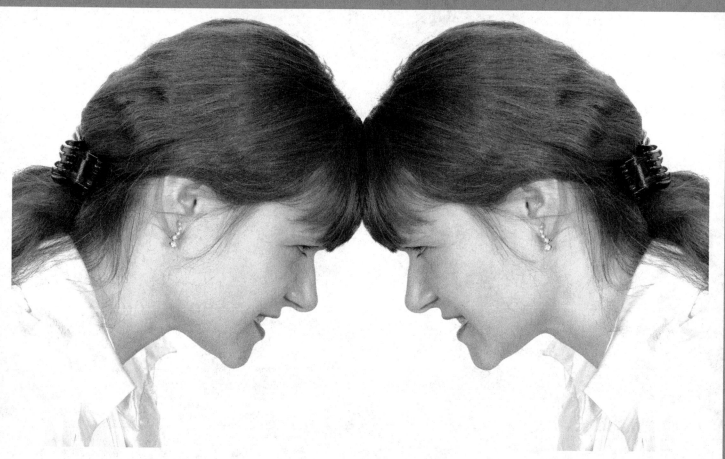

As far as she is concerned she is always right and has to have the last word. She has a lot of rules about how the world and people should be or not be. Never argue with an Aspie, I say. She struggles on a daily basis understanding that there are two ... no, three or more ... sides to a story and sometimes there can be as many perspectives as there are people!   —Younger sister of outspoken undiagnosed woman

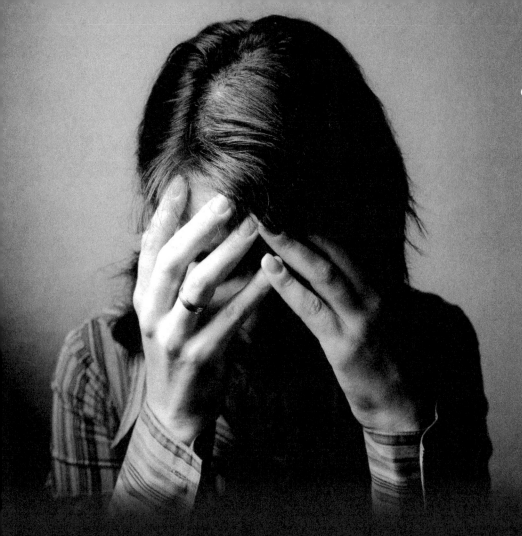

I had my first depression as a child and have battled with it, on and off, for most of my life. I am prone to depression attacks and now practise relapse prevention and extreme self-care daily to prevent any further episodes. Loneliness and isolation are hard for me.

She has a tendency to think negatively and then make decisions based on those thoughts. She tends to catastrophise ... even walked out on jobs ... she had a great opportunity literally handed to her, misunderstood her boss, catastrophised, then packed up her belongings and just took off. She couldn't face the truth, so she lied about the event. She owed her boss a whole bunch of money. She is now undergoing an assessment.

– Parents of intelligent 23-year-old with undiagnosed Autism

I can't socialise unless I am drinking or taking something to calm me down. I am so shy and it helps me manage my anxiety and stress. That's when I feel normal, relaxed and in control. I'm a recovering drug addict; you can't even tell I'm Autistic when I'm using drugs or drinking alcohol. I'm clean now and learning to manage my emotions and sensory issues in healthy ways.

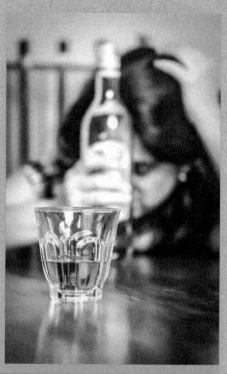

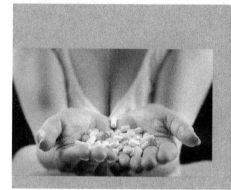

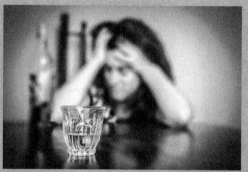

She is undiagnosed and blames others for her actions. She started drinking as a teenager. She says it helps her manage stress, stop the thoughts and be social. She has been doing this for years and we are struggling to find someone to help her and are really frustrated with the total lack of specialists in this area. We have been unable to get her the help she needs. She is enrolled in Dialectical Behavioural Training and modified Cognitive Behavioural Training classes which are helping her with the anxiety and stress, which is why she used in the first place.

– Sister of undiagnosed female on disability and in a day-treatment program

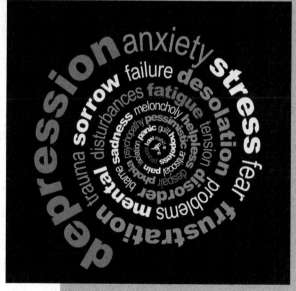

I literally cannot speak when others are angry with me, I mean I go mute. When I'm angry though, I have no trouble speaking! My temper has always been an issue for me, but people and life are just so frustrating.

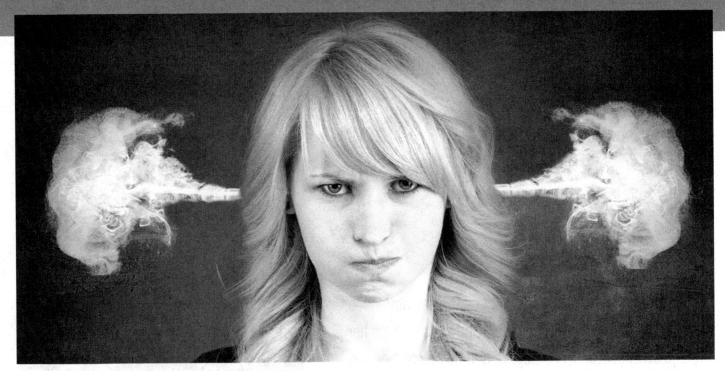

She has always had problems managing her strong emotions. She overreacts and goes to the extreme with people, then wonders why they don't want anything to do with her. In her mind, she thinks she is justified in her behaviours. She has a misguided sense of justice and can have terrible mood swings and lash out at people. She wants to be like other people; she wants to go out and do the same things that her peers are doing, but she can't do that. She is enraged about this and feels that life is not fair. She says she is dumb, despite her intelligence, has nothing to look forward to and self-harms daily. She will celebrate her 23rd birthday this year, yet she feels that there is no hope for her ever living a normal life. We are worried she will take her own life.

– Concerned parents looking for help

I just feel too much emotion to even speak about an issue. I explode, and I've lost jobs, lost contracts, lost writing and publishing deals, lost gigs, lost speaking opportunities. Everyone is out to get me.

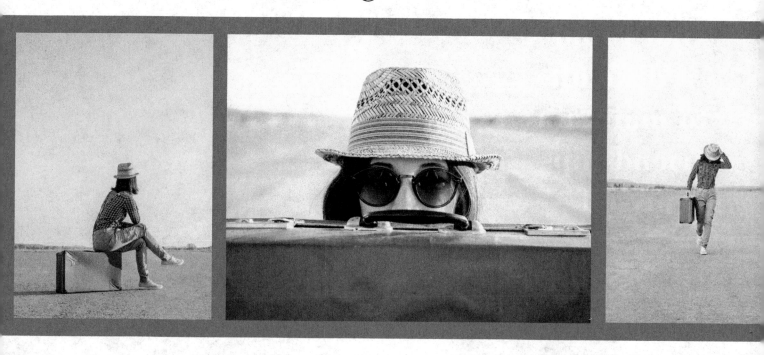

We assist females with emotion regulation and impulsivity, to learn to calm down and wait before reacting. The tendency to misinterpret and misperceive others coupled with anger, impulsiveness and lack of conflict resolution skills are some of their biggest struggles. There is a tendency to shoot first and ask questions later, which leaves others completely baffled. Learning more appropriate ways of handling conflict, including reparation skills, is crucial. Here at our centre we offer a range of programs including social skills training, assertiveness training, communication skills training and emotion regulation training. — Therapist and social worker

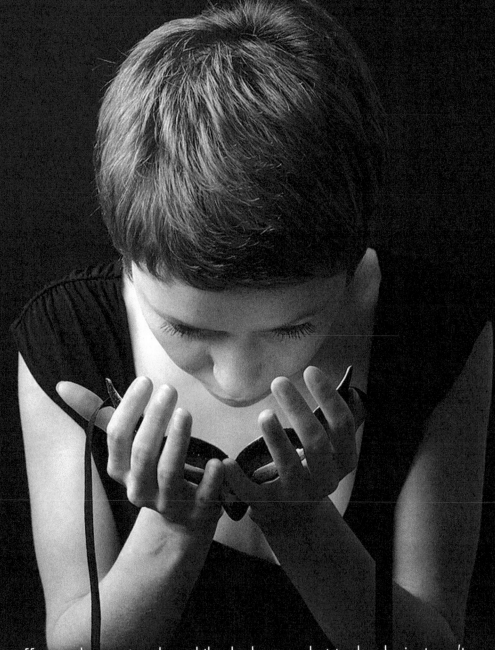

I am really interested in people and human behaviour but I find it difficult to maintain friendships myself.

She says they take so much time, effort and attention that while she knows what to do, she just can't do it. She spends so much energy and time masking her difficulties as it is.

— Parents of intelligent and socially exhausted undiagnosed 27-year-old

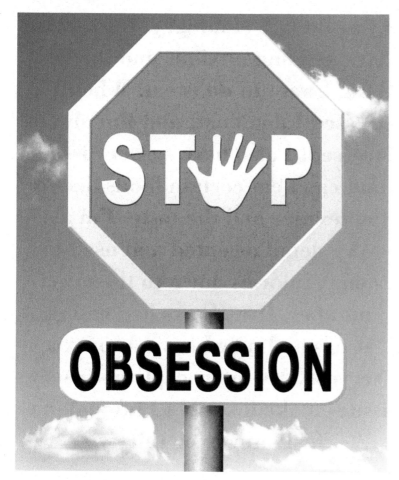

Throughout my life I have had intense interests: nature, animals, reading and books, technology and at times, other people. I have been in trouble with the police for being obsessive and stalking people.

At times throughout her life she has become obsessed with people and when that happens she finds it challenging to control. She has been involved with the law for stalking other people when she was younger.

– Social worker

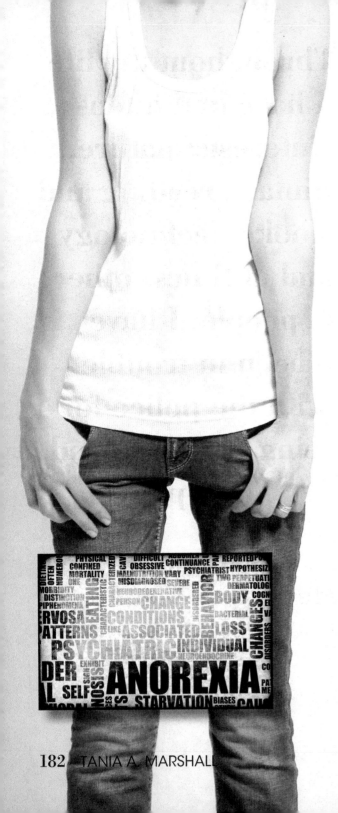

I just don't feel hungry. I'm always stressed and anxious and the last thing I want to do is eat. When I'm stressed I don't eat, and I'm always stressed! I also have sensory issues and can't eat certain foods due to the texture and the taste. I'm also very detail oriented and used to count calories down to the exact number. I've always had eating issues and now I have Anorexia Nervosa. My interoceptive sensory issues make it so that I often don't feel hungry or thirsty.

A screening program for all females who come into a clinic with an eating disorder is desperately needed. It is critical to know if a client has Autism or has symptoms of Autism because the symptoms were there from birth and are usually lifelong. The client may receive assistance for their eating disorder and the Autism goes unnoticed or untreated. Treating an eating disorder in a client with Autism is often different than treating a client with an eating disorder only.

– Psychiatrist

My executive function skills and sense of direction are shocking; I get lost all the time and have no idea where I am. It's extremely stressful.

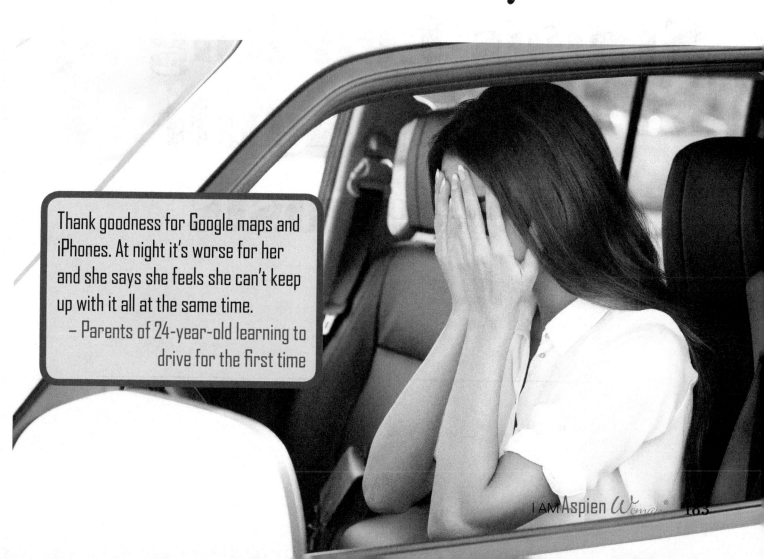

Thank goodness for Google maps and iPhones. At night it's worse for her and she says she feels she can't keep up with it all at the same time.
– Parents of 24-year-old learning to drive for the first time

Stages Leading up to an Adult Diagnosis

TANIA A. MARSHALL

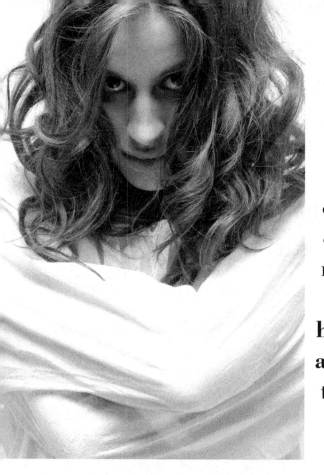

I am 50 years old and just received my diagnosis of adult female Autism.

I have been diagnosed with every label imaginable. Some of them were misdiagnoses, some were my ways of coping with Autism and some are a part or co-exist with my Autism. I have been restrained more times than I can count, locked up, on thorazine cocktails and had ECT. I remember trying to tell them about my sensory issues and they told me they thought I was schizophrenic. I then had a spectacular meltdown, which of course made me look even worse.

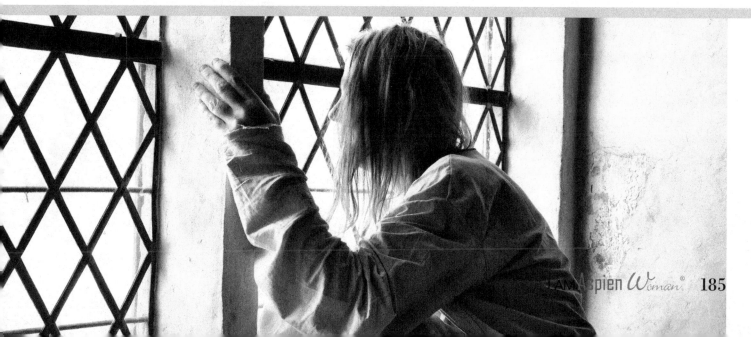

Many adult clients we see have a history of misdiagnosis, inappropriate treatment and often post-traumatic stress disorder. At that time the diagnosis of Autism or Asperger Syndrome did not exist. It was initially applied to males and is therefore a quite new explanation for the unique profile of females. It is not uncommon to hear that it "took me eight years and multiple diagnoses – bipolar type 2, borderline personality disorder, post-traumatic stress disorder, anxiety disorder – before I received my diagnosis of Autism".

– Psychologist

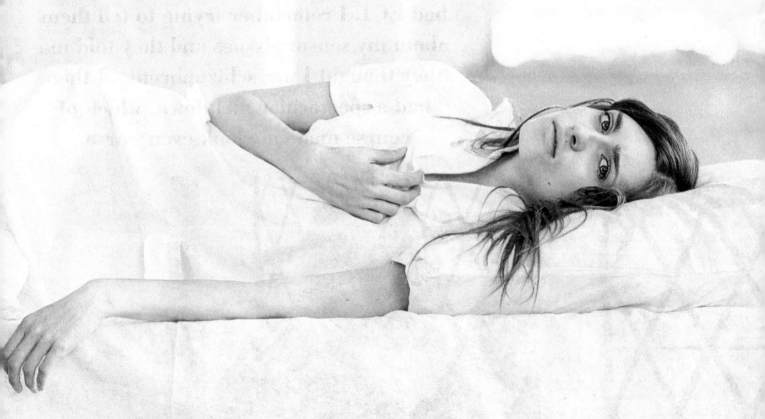

For as long as I remember I've been trying to figure myself out. I was first labelled as shy, and quiet. They told my parents I'd grow out of it.

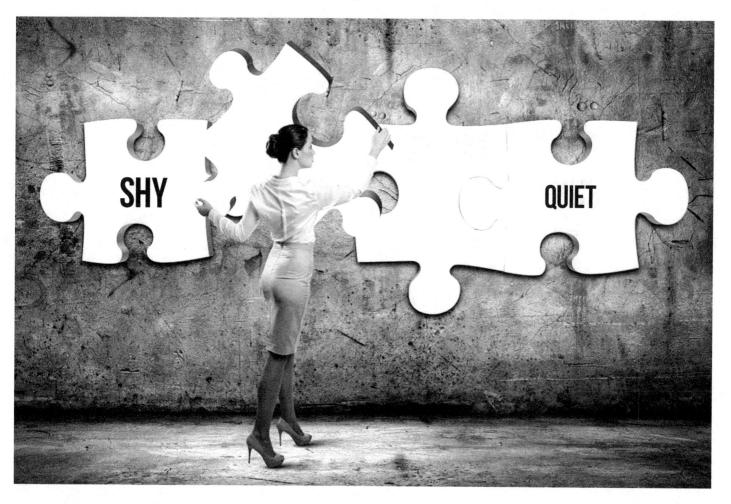

In reading hundreds of adult autobiographical descriptions, it is quite common for me to read the first descriptions of self to include: "shyness", "social anxiety", "a daydreamer", and/or "played on my own".

– Tania A. Marshall, psychologist

Then came the labels Attention Deficit Hyperactivity Disorder (ADHD) and social anxiety

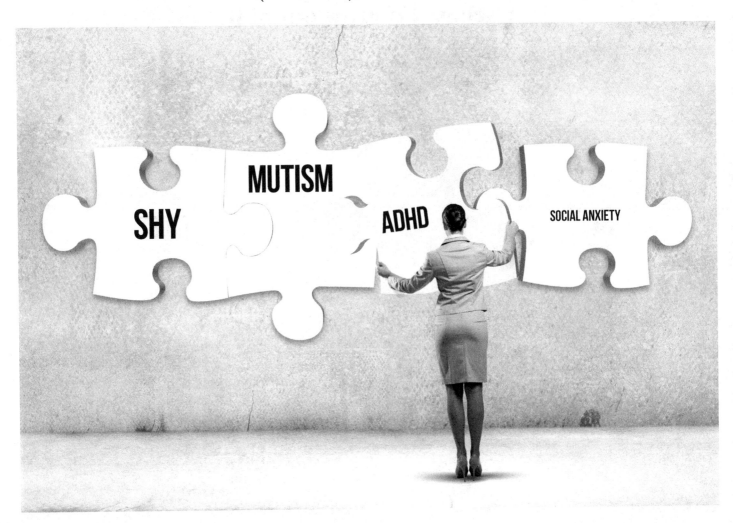

Further along the autobiographical description, another theme that is common is that the client may have had a suggestion or diagnosis of ADHD and anxiety disorder.

– Tania A. Marshall, psychologist

In my teen years, I was very depressed, had a nervous breakdown and an eating disorder.

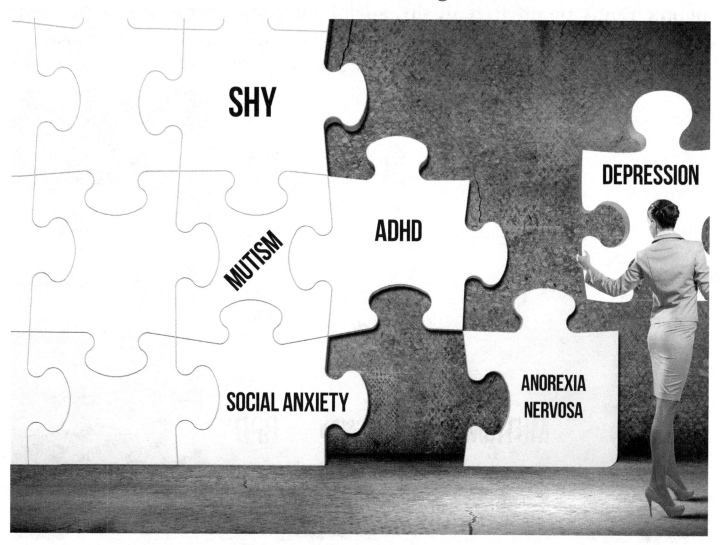

SHY

MUTISM

ADHD

DEPRESSION

SOCIAL ANXIETY

ANOREXIA NERVOSA

Common teenage experiences include a nervous breakdown or depressive episode with many females also saying they had either eating issues or an eating disorder, as an older child or teenager.

– Tania A. Marshall, psychologist

Then came additional labels of bipolar disorder, borderline personality disorder traits and post-traumatic stress disorder. Can people really be intelligent, shy, socially anxious, mute and depressed bipolar anorexics with borderline personality disorder and post-traumatic stress disorder?!

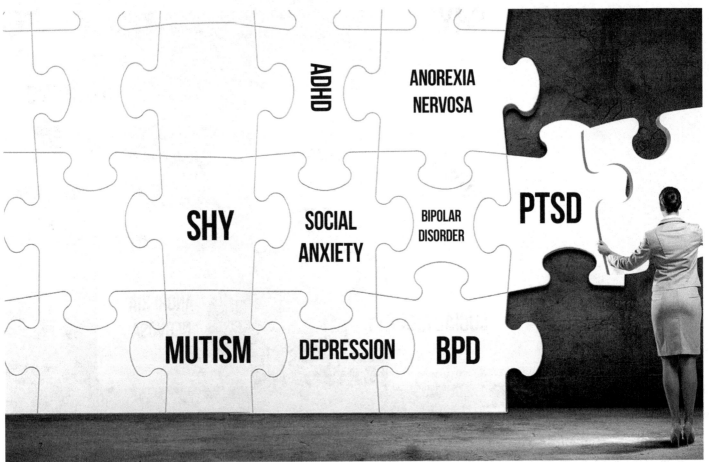

A common theme in the autobiographies reveals a long history of counselling, attending psychologist, psychiatrist appointments, individual or group therapy, inpatient and/or outpatient visits and many diagnoses, some appropriate and some not appropriate.

– Tania A. Marshall, psychologist

I have had just about every label in existence, including schizophrenia. Recently, I received a diagnosis of epilepsy.

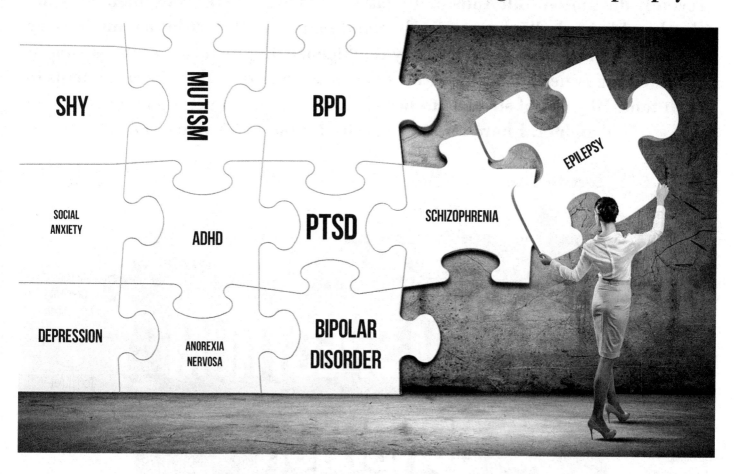

SHY

MUTISM

BPD

SOCIAL ANXIETY

ADHD

PTSD

SCHIZOPHRENIA

EPILEPSY

DEPRESSION

ANOREXIA NERVOSA

BIPOLAR DISORDER

A common theme running through the autobiographical descriptions from females is one of receiving many different diagnoses and/or being misdiagnosed. Some women have been misdiagnosed with schizophrenia, borderline personality disorder or another personality. Some women do have both Autism and a co-existing personality disorder, which is a very complex presentation for professionals, their families and other support workers to understand and challenging to live with.

– Tania A. Marshall, psychologist

I read about Asperger Syndrome but felt that it didn't fit. I then came across female Autism and it fit me like a glove. It explained my daughter who is recently diagnosed with Autism, my father who was an engineer, memories of school and being bullied to very public and magnificent meltdowns, my sensory sensitivities and social difficulties, my intelligence despite a lack of it showing in school, eating issues, difficulties with stress and anxiety and my savant talents in art. It took 10 years of struggle to be taken seriously and get a diagnosis for my daughter. I have now just received mine at 66 years old.

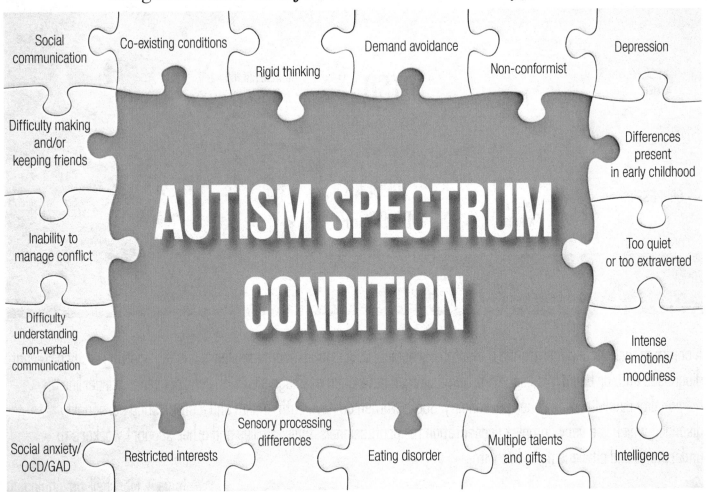

After the diagnosis, I felt like I was 'born again'. I felt immense relief, I then felt anger (anger that "if they had known back then" … but of course they didn't know back then what Autism was). I feel much less like a 'weirdo' and more like a person who is wired differently and that feels good. I would like to be me, although I don't know who that is. It's never too late for an adult diagnosis and there are far more advantages to gaining one than not, at any age.

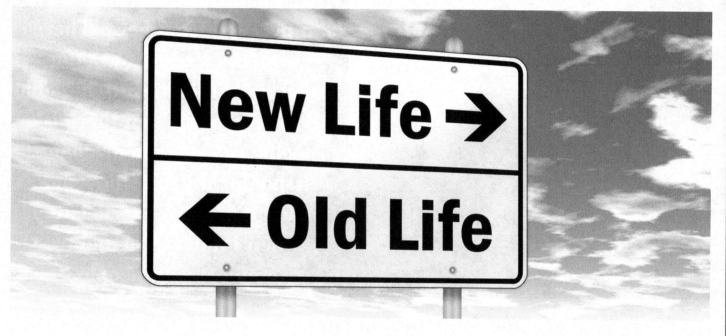

As a part of an 'assessment' I include a 'What Next?' section, covering knowledge and awareness of the diagnosis, education and referring to information and/or research related to female Autism, having a strengths-based attitude, addressing challenges, discussion of work, educational or career options, addressing parenting or motherhood. This is tailored to each individual person based on their unique situation, their age, any co-existing conditions or disorders, and where they present in terms of severity of characteristics (social, communication, emotional, sensory, relationship and interests). We also work on starting a strengths list, a 'Who Am I?' workbook and a sensory profile and sensory management kit.

– Tania A. Marshall, psychologist and author

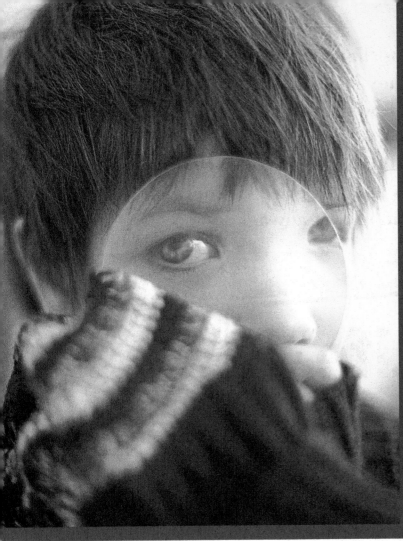

Autism for me was a new lens to look through, giving me the awareness, self-understanding and education about how my brain works, what kind of a thinker I am, what my strengths (and challenges) are and where to proceed from here. There was a deep sense of shame about my difficulties. Being able to say to people that there is a specific reason (a neurological issue) for my weirdness has made it feel less excruciating when I don't fit in and or connect with people.

I include in my 'What Next?' section a discussion around some possible future experience with family members, friends or co-workers. Many well-meaning people may not believe the client or invalidate her struggles and/or diagnosis. Post-diagnostic support helps to prepare the client to cope and manage with people not understanding that females present differently than males. Supporting the client in how to respond when people say, "You?! You have Autism? But you can look at me? But you can have a conversation with me?" or "You don't look like you have Autism", is an important part of post-diagnosis support.

– Tania A. Marshall, psychologist and author

I used to blame myself a lot for not being able to socialise or manage my time or multi-task, or go to the grocery shops, or eat certain foods. Now I understand why some things are so hard for me and other things are really easy for me. I reframed my life experiences and was able to forgive myself, not be so hard on myself, accept what I can't do, focus on what I can do and my partner and family understand me better. At 39, I feel like I have finally grown up and am ready to start being an adult.

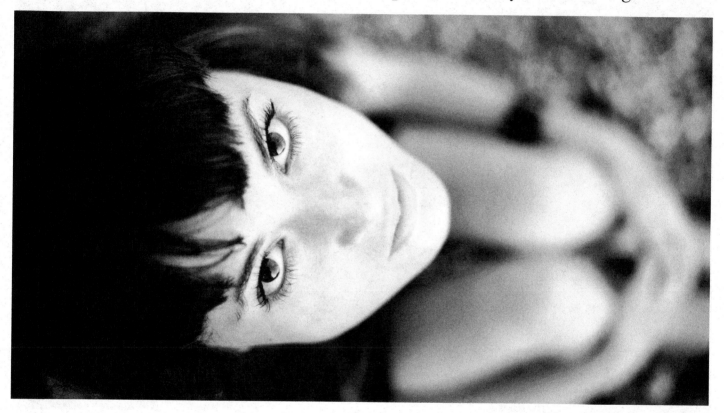

It can take some time for clients to work through a late diagnosis. A reframing process is usually quite helpful in terms of awareness and answers of past experiences and self-understanding. An important topic to discuss is the exploration of interests, talents, gifts and strengths, in addition to addressing challenges. A positive and strengths-based attitude is a must.

– Tania A. Marshall, psychologist and author

It really wasn't until I understood myself and my experiences, learnt what my strengths are and nurtured them, addressed my challenges, received support and help, and made environmental and academic accommodations, that life became easier for me. The diagnosis was the starting place for me. I always dabbled in art, but now two years later, I am a successful painter.

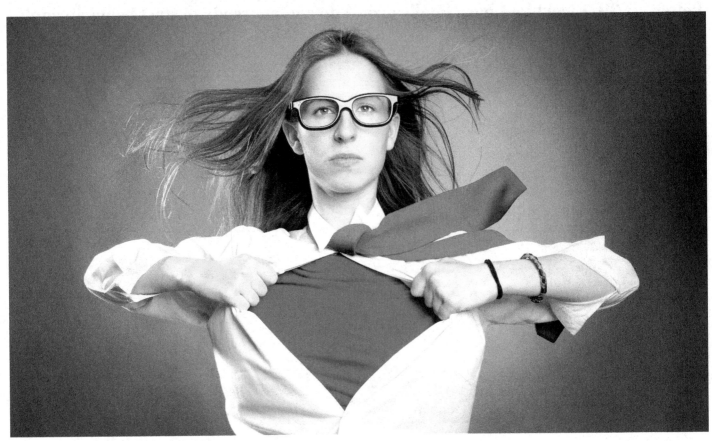

I have found that they tend to function best when they have had a formal diagnosis, understand what type of thinker they are, understand their unique profile of strengths/gifts and weaknesses, are actively involved and using their strengths and gifts, maintain a calm inner and outer world, practise extreme self-care, and most importantly, have understanding, flexible and supportive people in their lives.

- Tania A. Marshall, psychologist

Important Aspien-Woman Needs

I cannot be myself or function well when I am constrained by 'the box'. I think and learn differently than my peers. Please let me out of the box.

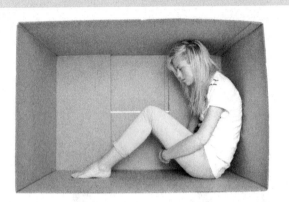 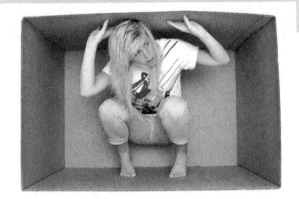

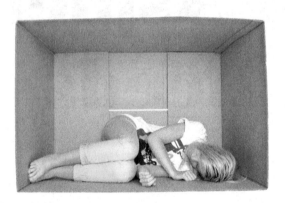 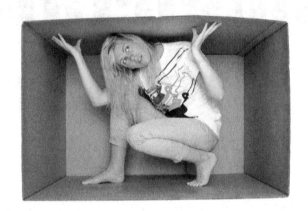

Here at our school we have many students who are 'out of the box' thinkers. Individuals on the spectrum perceive the world differently and many have great difficulty in regular mainstream schools. Many of the students here are at risk of dropping out and our school was created for these individuals. She needs more time or less work, is at different grade levels in terms of her academic subjects and has a great need to teach herself. She receives academic accommodations, social skills training and relaxation training, She is much happier and on her way to graduating.

– School psychologist of Year 12 student private special needs school

Please give me space and solitude. I need it like I need to breathe air. Quiet periods of time restore me emotionally. I need help learning how to implement extreme self-care, so that I don't burn out every so often. I need to have a calm internal (body and brain) and external environment (home, work, school). I have all kinds of disappearing tricks which help me manage a social hangover.

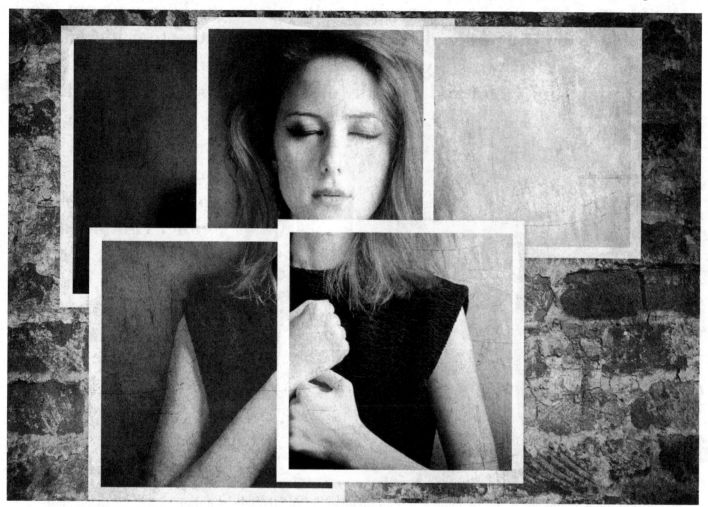

Extreme self-care means getting to know oneself first. Having an understanding of one's own unique nervous system and how much socialising, activity, work and demands an individual can manage, without burning out. Practising daily relaxation, getting physical exercise, getting enough solitude, and staying on a schedule is vital. Since she reduced her social cup, she has more energy.

– Social worker

Please try to understand and accept my differences. I was born different. I didn't come with the handbook of social rules and socialising is not my strong point. My facial expressions may not match my emotions, my tone of voice may not be appropriate to the situation. They may not even be related to my emotional state. I am highly sensitive to criticism so please present it very gently. I misinterpret others often. I'm a serious person who thinks a lot and I usually mean no disrespect. My condition is not an excuse, but an explanation. I'm sure I am allergic to conflict because I will either run the other way, avoiding it at all possible costs, or I just explode. I have learnt that this is not a good strategy and plan to learn assertiveness training.

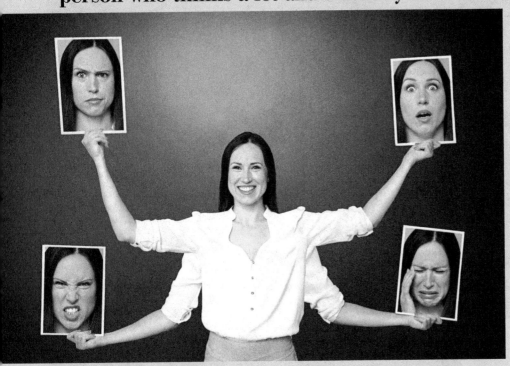

After fighting for a diagnosis, many females are then faced with the struggle of obtaining acknowledgement and validation and are desperate to be believed, even within the Autistic community. A client told me that even other Autistic people have trouble believing her and the worst part for her is that her superior blending skills have compensated for her difficulties and she sometimes feels she does not belong anywhere. They need acknowledgement of their struggles and validation of their diagnosis. – Tania A. Marshall, psychologist

I need to go step by step at my own pace or I can get easily stressed. I need more time to process information, think about and make decisions (little or big), complete tasks or coursework. I love to teach myself and I am usually really good at it. I may need help with paperwork, filling out forms and organisation.

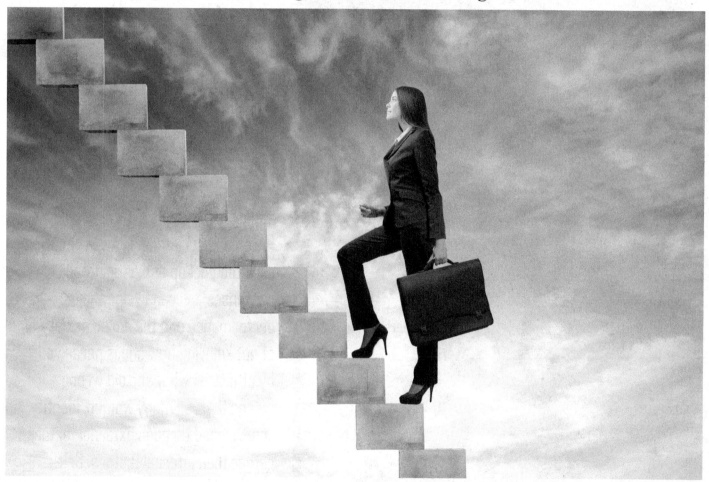

She is very good at her work, but has a tendency to get quite overwhelmed by too many demands placed on her, deadlines, pressure and/or too much work ... even her perception of too much can cause her stress and worry.

– Disability services support worker

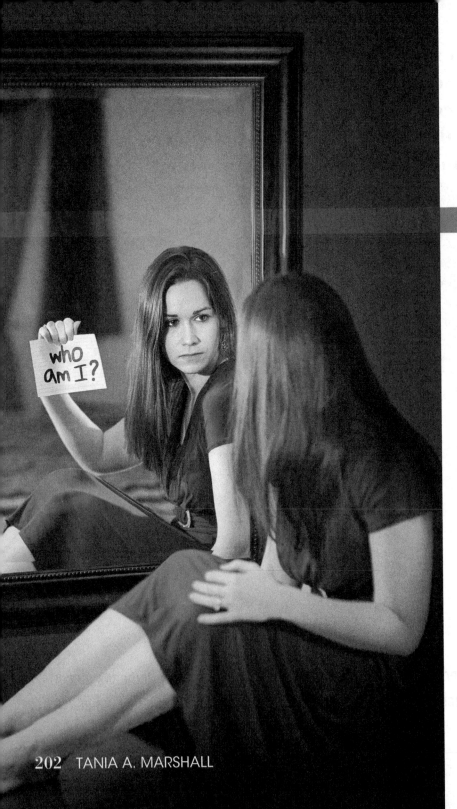

I have practised the parts of other people my whole life; I have no idea of who I am, no identity or self-esteem.

Self-esteem, identity and the question 'who am I?' has great meaning for women with Autism. Having lived their lives as chameleons and practising social echolalia like award-winning actresses, there is a price to pay. Practising scripts and lines, preparing scripted backup and anticipated responses, overanalysing their performance and the added anxiety of not knowing how she is perceived by others or what she did wrong means that for many women, identity is developed through external factors rather than internal factors. Self-esteem, identity work and exploring strengths is vital for their mental health.

– Tania A. Marshall, psychologist and author

Teach me how to think in more helpful, more positive and more flexible ways. I think in black and white, all or nothing thinking.

Flexibility of thinking and seeing the shades of grey is something she has worked very hard on and it has helped her relationship with others enormously. She is a real self-improvement guru.

— Aunt of self-improvement expert

Allow me to make accommodations to my home, school and/or work environments to assist me with my sensory processing issues. My psychologist worked with me to understand my unique sensory profile and helped me develop my own sensory coping kit, which goes with me everywhere. I have headphones, ear plugs, sunglasses, hat, my bottle of lavender, my necklace (with a ceramic bottle I put calming essential oils into), a scarf and my iPod.

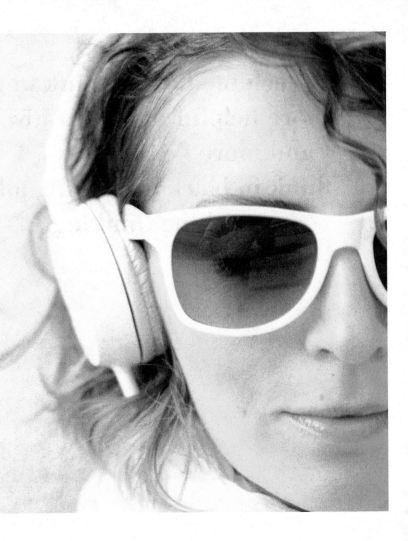

The creation of sensory management kits are crucial for every individual with Autism or Asperger Syndrome. Each individual has a unique sensory processing style and it is highly beneficial for them to understand their unique sensory profile and how to manage their sensory differences.   – Occupational therapist

Help me to learn how to manage my emotions and learn to tolerate distress.

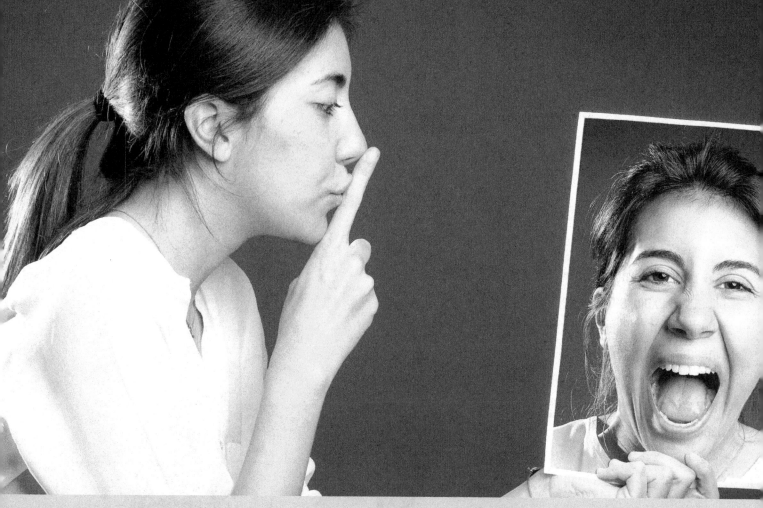

Learning about body clues, triggers and stressors, unhelpful thinking styles, sensory issues, extreme self-care skills, emotions and emotion regulations skills, in addition to modifications to the environment, can all help to improve distress tolerance. — Therapist working with people with emotion dysregulation

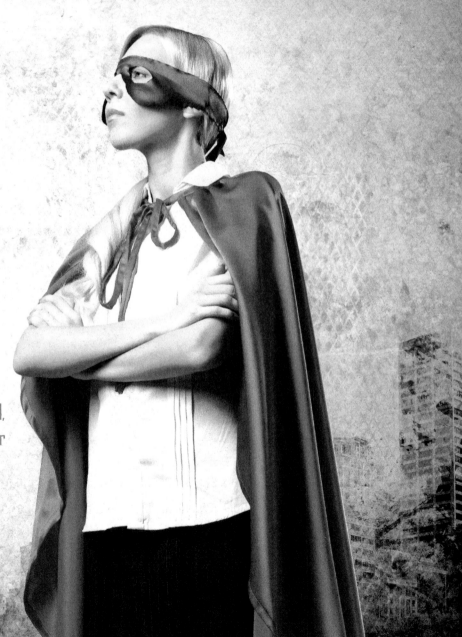

Please help me discover and pursue my strengths, gifts and talents for it is this that makes me happy and gives me a sense of purpose and meaning.

A large part of my work involves helping clients to explore their areas of strength, what type of thinker they may be, and where they would like to go from here in terms of their future. Many females have so many talents they have trouble deciding!

– Tania A. Marshall,
psychologist and author

It is never too late to receive a diagnosis. With the right diagnosis and support many AspienWomen are known to fly; we can be our own superheros, the best versions of ourselves.

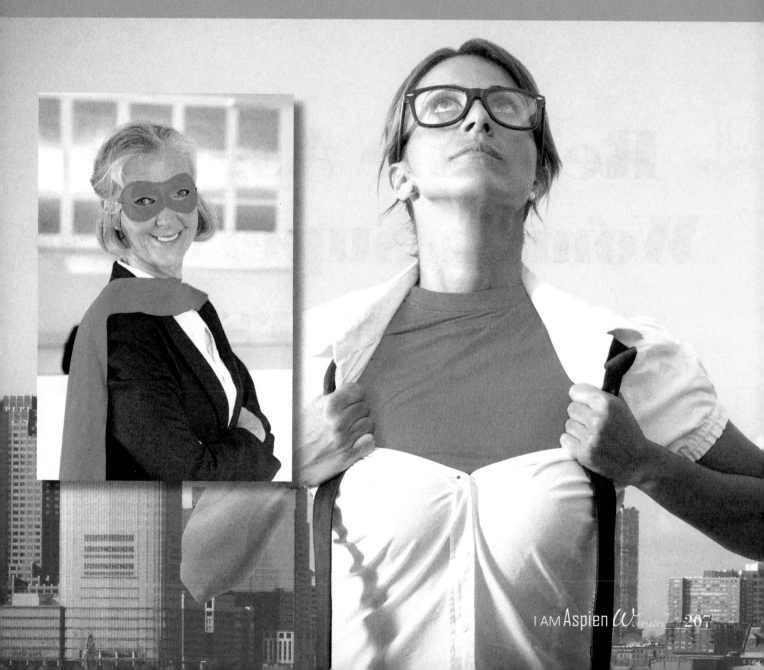

Real-life Aspien-Woman Superhero Mentors

TANIA A. MARSHALL

Dr Temple Grandin

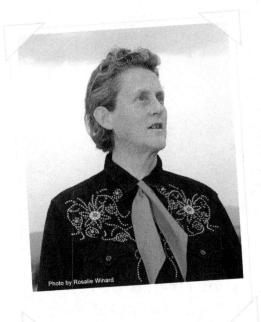

Photo by Rosalie Winard

I am Dr Temple Grandin, aged 67, diagnosed with Autism at age four

Professor of Animal Science, Colorado State University, USA

My Strengths:

1. Good at art and my art ability was always encouraged

2. You have to learn to be less rigid. Early in my career I learned it was better to get 80% of what I wanted and actually achieve it. Going for 100% was going to fail

3. An early mentor told me that I was too negative and critical and I took his advice. This helped my career

4. Thinking in pictures, working with animals, writing, and intelligence

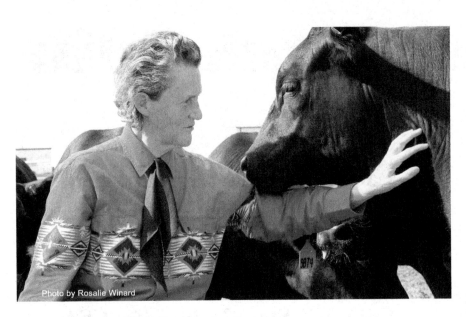

Photo by Rosalie Winard

My Top Tips:

1. Find good mentors who will help you develop your strengths. I can't emphasise enough the value of mentors for others. I had a great science teacher as a mentor and I had mentors in the cattle industry who recognised my abilities. In my work as a professor, I have mentored many students and I have opened the door for several students who may have been mildly on the Autism spectrum. One of my mentors at the Swift Meat Plant in the 1970s said, "You always have to persevere." Mentors can be found in many unexpected places.

2. Mentors may actively find you if they know about your work. A building contractor who was an important mentor actually sought my services. He guided me on getting my design career started.

3. Make a portfolio of your best work. People respect ability.

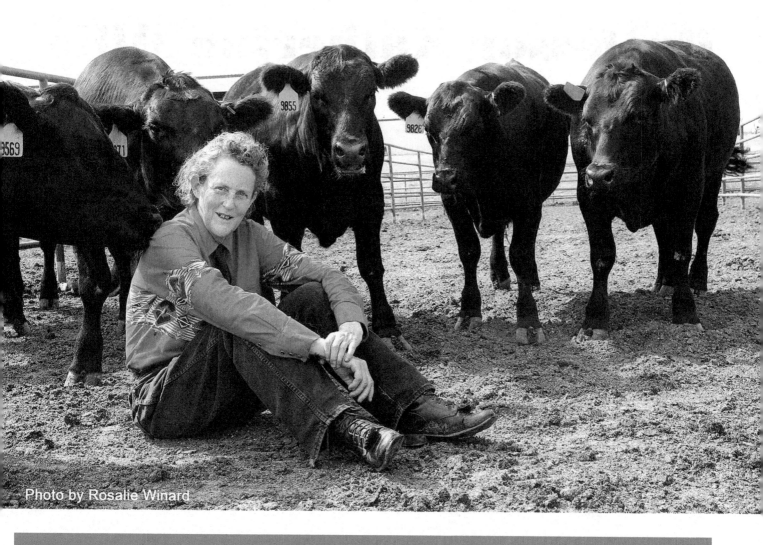

Photo by Rosalie Winard

Temple can be reached or followed at:
W: http://www.templegrandin.com
T: @DrTempleGrandin
F: https://www.facebook.com/drtemplegrandin

Professor Katherine Milla

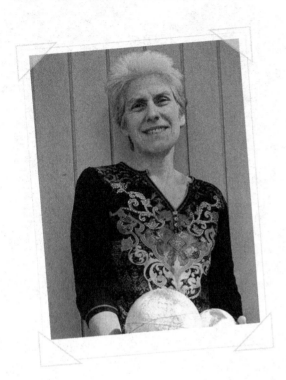

I am Professor Katherine Milla, aged 53, diagnosed with Asperger Syndrome at age 51

Geologist, professor, photographer, Aspie life coach, USA

My Strengths (aka, survival skills):

1. Improvising (MacGyver style)

2. Perceptiveness

3. Finding the path of least resistance

4. Ninja-style stealth, shape-shifting and artful passive-aggression in the service of minimising conflict

5. Sense of humour

My Top Tips:

1. If you feel like you are the only one of your species, then you are the only one who can teach you how to be you. Take notes, study well and do your homework.

2. Make a kind and loving space for your fear, but don't let her drive.

3. I discovered my place on the spectrum at 51. Since then I have struggled with regrets over my life choices, grief for lost opportunities and anger over the missed diagnosis. These are natural feelings that must be honoured. Then accept that one cannot move forward while looking backward. Choosing one path necessarily means that there are many you must walk away from. Choose anyway. Take your compass, learn to read it, and trust it. It will lead you where you need to be.

**Katherine can be reached:
E: aslifecoach@protonmail.com**

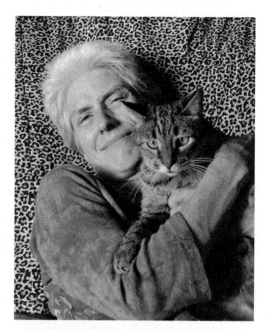

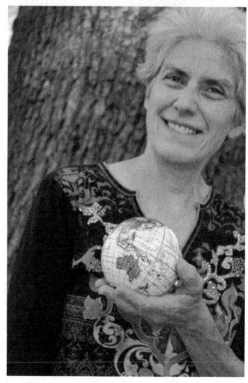

Lauren Lovejoy

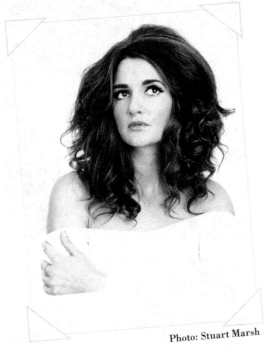

Photo: Stuart Marsh

I am Lauren Lovejoy, aged 25, diagnosed with Asperger Syndrome at age 14

Professional singer, songwriter, model and actress, UK

National Autistic Society (NAS) Ambassador, UK

Miss Universe Great Britain, 'Miss Congeniality'and Miss 'Not in Vein' Awards

My Strengths:

1. Singing and song writing

2. Writing poetry, modelling

3. Making people laugh

4. Making a difference and being a positive ambassador for Autistic Nottingham and Children's Strong Bones charity and now a National Autistic Society (NAS) Ambassador.

5. I am a great believer in positive thinking. I admit there have been times in my life when I have not wanted to be around anymore; however, what you have to think is there is always going to be someone else in the world worse off than you, keep strong and positive, and this will inspire others like ourselves to do the same. This attitude has made me a much happier and more confident person today. I have helped inspire others to overcome their obstacles; the people I have inspired say they feel they now have more confidence to achieve what they want to in life. As long as I can make others happy that is all what matters

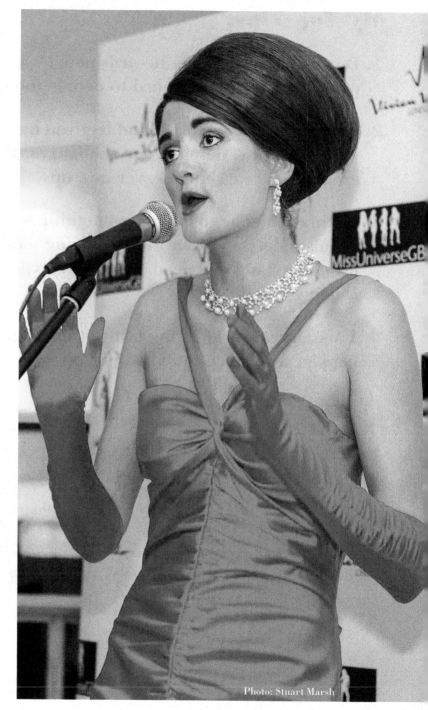

Photo: Stuart Marsh

My Top Tips:

1. Do not be too trusting towards people you meet straight away. Some Autistic people tend to get attached to people too quickly. Learn about boundaries.

2. Try not to give up in life and feel you have a barrier in front of you. Focus on your strengths, despite your challenges. Being Autistic makes us even more creative and we should never give up.

3. Asking someone to explain something to you if you misunderstand something or misunderstand what you are being told to do. Some Autistic people can misunderstand and need alternative explanations in order to understand what is being asked.

4. I am a great believer in positive thinking. This attitude has made me a much happier and more confident person today.

Lauren can be reached or followed at:
T: @laurenlovejoy6
F: www.facebook.com/laurenlovejoyofficial
You can listen to Lauren on SoundCloud:
W: https://soundcloud.com/lauren-lovejoy

Jeanette Purkis

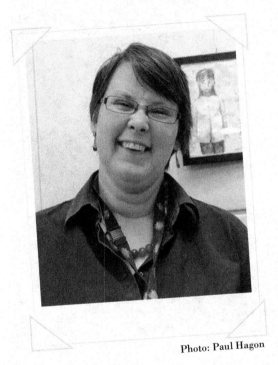

Photo: Paul Hagon

I am Jeanette Purkis, aged 40, diagnosed with Asperger Syndrome at age 20 in 1994

Author, presenter, Autism advocate and public servant, Australia

My Strengths:

1. Creativity
2. Determination
3. Kindness and compassion
4. Intelligence
5. I can write anything
6. Animal empath

My Top Tips:

1. Where you're at now is not necessarily where you will be in the future. We don't know what's down the track and it might just be wonderful. When I was 25 I was a homeless ex-prisoner. Now I'm an internationally published author, career public servant and Autism advocate.

2. Don't doubt yourself. You are amazing. Just think how much you've come through, dealt with and mastered over your lifetime.

3. Meet, befriend, and spend time with healthy people – especially women – on the spectrum. They are a great peer group, support network and source of fun and laughter. The first time I was in a room full of other AspienWomen I felt like I had come home.

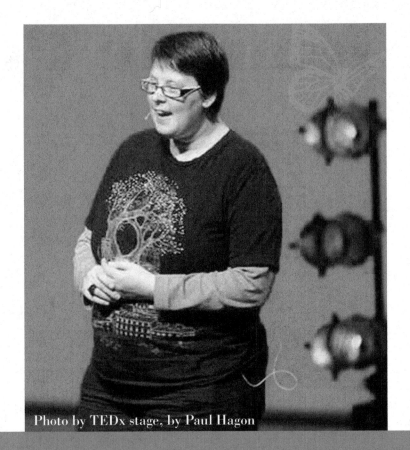

Photo by TEDx stage, by Paul Hagon

Jeanette can be reached or followed at:

The Jeanette Purkis Women's Group is a group I run through the Autism Asperger ACT www.autismaspergeract.com.au/our-services/the-jeanette-purkis-women-s-group

People who are interested in attending can also contact me via email on jeanettepurkis@gmail.com

T: @jeanettepurkis

F: www.facebook.com/jeanettepurkisbooks

Olley Edwards

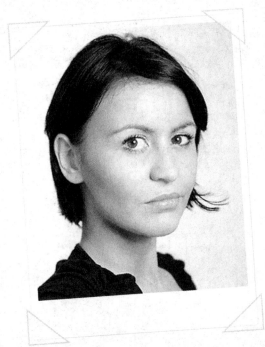

I am Olley Edwards, aged 33, diagnosed with Asperger Syndrome at age 32, 2015 at the Lorna Wing Centre, Bromley UK

Filmmaker and director, script writer, author of *Why Aren't Normal People Normal?*, Autism advocate

Olley also attended and spoke on female Autism at the World Human Rights Forum in Marrakesh, 2014

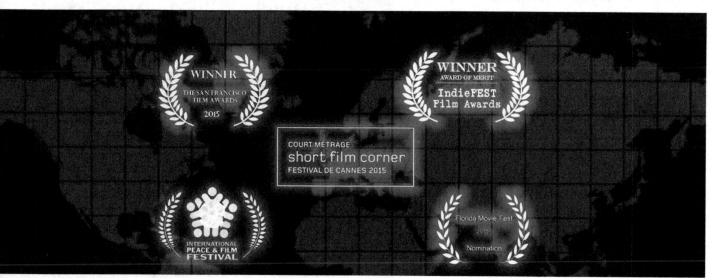

My Strengths:

1. Creative thinking
2. Film making
3. Determination

My Top Tips:

1. Understand your natural vulnerability and naivety and learn how to protect yourself. You have to learn how and when to set boundaries and how to keep safe.

2. Learn to logically and non-emotively look at the condition you have and learn how to help yourself in certain areas.

3. Do not expect that everyone with the same diagnosis will be the same as you are. Even though we are all on the spectrum, we are all different from each other. We are unique, and have different personality traits.

Olley can be reached or followed at:
T: @olleyedwards
Epidemic of Knowledge Movie
W: www.epidemicofknowledge.com/
http://film.britishcouncil.org/
epidemic-of-knowledge
W: www.facebook.com/
EpidemicOfKnowledge
T: @eokaspergers

The Kindest Label Movie
ANACA award for visual arts, available for viewing at:
https://www.youtube.com/
watch?v=Ctn6uBmUVgk

Why Aren't Normal People Normal? Book
Available at Amazon: http://www.
amazon.com/Why-Arent-Normal-
People-ebook/dp/B00F5WA47M

Jen Saunders

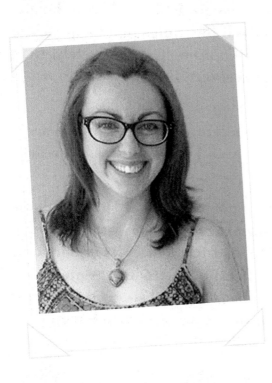

I am Jen Saunders, aged 27, diagnosed with Asperger Syndrome at age 26

Successful entrepreneur, Australia

My Strengths:

1. **Writing:** I've only been writing for a few years, but it has changed my life. I have trouble expressing my feelings verbally, and in that sense, writing has saved me

2. **Creativity:** I've always loved to draw, paint and design

3. **Hyperfocus:** this allows me to 'get in the zone' when I'm working on something I'm passionate about

4. **Empathy + sensitivity:** While it can sometimes be intense and I'm not always able to express it, I'm very sensitive. I have a lot of empathy for others, particularly animals, children and women

My Top Tips:

1. When I first realised I could be Aspie, I went through a whole range of emotions. I went through a period of grieving, of letting go of the life I thought I 'should' have. I came out the other side feeling positive. I was able to forgive myself for things that happened in the past. I was able to see the positive of being Aspie and embrace it completely. In fact, being diagnosed gave me the freedom to let go of the pressure I'd always felt to try to fit in.

2. Telling others or not is entirely your choice. I chose to tell my family and even share my story on my blog, but I have a very supportive family so I knew they would react positively.

3. Surround yourself with people who are healthy and support you. After sharing about my diagnosis on my blog, I received tons of emails from other AspienWomen who could relate to everything I said, and it felt so good to chat to others who understood me. That's why I co-founded the Autistic Women's Collective, to create a community for women on the spectrum and foster understanding, support and sisterhood. There's something so validating and liberating about sharing your story and then having someone say "I thought I was the only one who thought/felt that way."

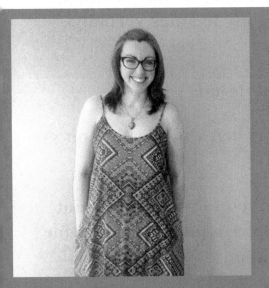

Jen can be reached or followed at:
Founder + CEO
Wild Sister Magazine
W: www.wildsister.com
Autistic Womens Collective
W: http://autisticwomenscollective.com

Chou Chou Scantlin

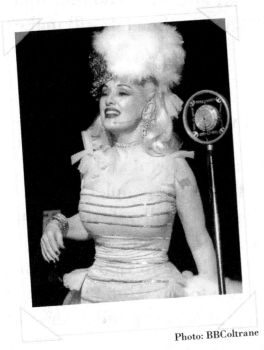

Photo: BBColtrane

I am Chou Chou Scantlin, aged 60, diagnosed with Autism at age 3

Professional singer, actress, and model, USA

Doc Scantlin Imperial Palms Orchestra

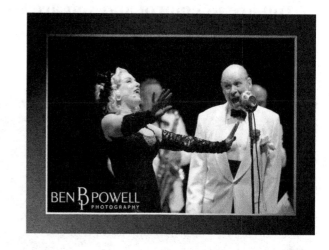

My Strengths:

1. Producer

2. Performer

3. Costumer

4. 'Queen of DIY'

5. My greatest gift of all? Being happy, because I learned that happiness is finding your gift and giving it away

My Top Tips:

1. Embrace your unique individuality and create a lifestyle that makes you thrive. You are not like most people. Embrace that, love that, and find what you have to give and give it, with all you've got! That, in the end, will make you happy with how you lived your life.

2. Above all, take care of yourself. Self-advocate and take the needed time to recover and recharge. Know what you need help with and ask for it.

3. Learn to see the best in yourself and others. We all are awful and do bad things, but are wonderful, too. I find it very hard to 'read' people, so I learned to assume they are charming and wonderful. Usually, if treated that way, people will try to prove me right. I guard myself from any potentially dangerous situations, but such things are rare if you learn to value the beauty and kindness in most of the people you run into day to day. Don't be a victim. You are in control and you are stronger than you think! To quote a very old, mostly forgotten song: 'It's a great life, if you don't give in!'

Chou Chou can be reached or followed at:
T: @docscantlin
Doc Scantlin & His Imperial Palms Orchestra
W: www.docscantlin.com
For booking information contact:
Chou Chou at Chou Chou Productions, LLC at: 410-535-6255
chouchou@docscantlin.com

In Memory of Laura Golden

(April 29, 1976 - September 20, 2014)

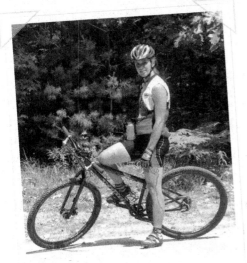

Photo: Deborah Chamberlain

I am Laura Golden, aged 38, undiagnosed Autism Spectrum Condition

Artist and cyclist, USA

My Strengths:

1. Artist, photographic memory, cyclist

2. Ghost/animal/plant whisperer

3. Atypical sense of humour and my explosive laugh

4. Unique reinvention of the English language

My Top Tips:

1. Do the things you love

2. Find and create space daily to recharge from all the overstimulation

3. There is a place for all of us in this world

Dedication to Laura

To my dear Laura,

My adventure-mate and friend extraordinaire, I met you on the Wendell Common at Old Home Day during the summer of 2008. You came into my life in a time of transition and pain. You brought to me a sense of calmness, stability, a level of attentiveness I was unaccustomed to. In your words, "Thank you for your love, adventure, play, gardening, exercising, and encouraging one another, sharing sobriety and many more … As each season passes, I am reminded of how deeply our lives were connected.

Love Deborah

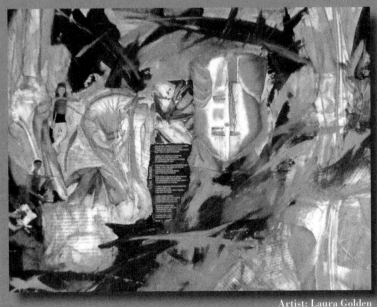

Artist: Laura Golden

Chelsea Hopkins-Allan

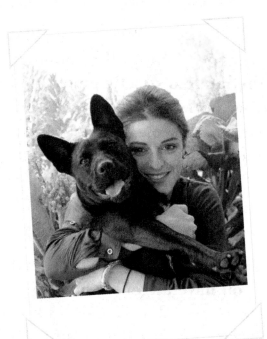

This is my dog Django and I in front of my vegetable garden.

I am Chelsea Hopkins-Allan, aged 27, diagnosed with Asperger Syndrome at age 19

Environmental scientist and artist, Australia

My Strengths:

1. Extremely determined, intelligent, independent

2. Compassionate + I care deeply about others and the state of community/the world

3. Friendly and outgoing, loyal

4. Creative and passionate about my interests

My Top Tips: (These are things I've learnt the hard way through experience!)

1: Eat clean

The Asperger-body seems to be a VERY finely tuned machine. If I could go back in time I would tell myself to change my diet and go strictly gluten and dairy free; limit caffeine, sugar and alcohol; avoid packaged and processed foods (even the gluten-free products); read labels and eat lots of raw veggies and some good fats. Your gut health has a huge impact on your brain functioning.

2: Trust your own judgement

As a woman with Asperger's you have almost certainly made frequent social mistakes with friends, family and others where you have angered, hurt or offended them unintentionally with a lack of interpersonal awareness. I know I sure have! Trust your own feelings and judgement in your relationships in spite of your challenges, even if you cannot identify the reason straight away. You might not know as much as others about all the interpersonal and social details but this does not make you automatically wrong about all things in your interactions with others. Do not doubt your ability to make your own decisions, stand up for what is morally right, set healthy boundaries for yourself or assert yourself.

3: Learn how to be a better conversationalist (and not lecture people on your special interests!)

Having a few simple and logical strategies to help with social and interpersonal interaction can go a long way.

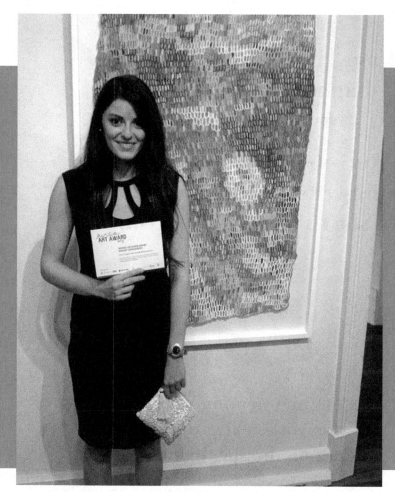

I paint modern Australian environmental science and mindfulness-inspired watercolour, gouache and mixed-media paintings.

Chelsea can be reached or followed at:
E: ChelseaHAart@gmail.com
F: www.facebook.com/ChelseaHopkinsAllanArt
I: @chelseahopkinsallan_art
Chelsea's art can be purchased from:
W: www.chelseah-a.com

Maja Toudal

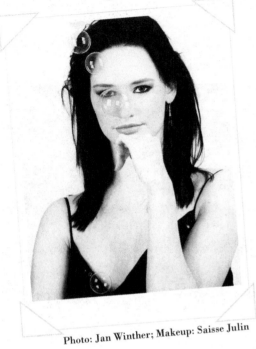

Photo: Jan Winther; Makeup: Saisse Julin

I am Maja Toudal, aged 28, diagnosed with Asperger Syndrome at age 16

Autism consultant, singer/ songwriter, Autism advocate, YouTuber (TheAnMish), Denmark.

My Strengths:

1. Expression through songwriting/ poetry and singing

2. Honesty (self-reflection)

3. Loyalty in friendship

4. Communicating with NTs (neurotypicals are people who are not on the spectrum)

5. Stubbornness in achieving goals

6. Focus when doing something I love/ special interest

My Top Tips:

1. Those who won't accept you are not worth your time or love. Allow yourself to live without them.

2. Some people will tell you (and you might tell yourself) that your diagnosis means there are things you can't do. Don't accept this as truth as it's amazing what we can do and learn over time. It might take a decade, but you'll get there, so keep fighting.

3. Accept that you will make many mistakes in your life, and view each one as an opportunity to learn. It's not the end of the world, it's a chance to improve.

6. Focus when doing something I love/special interest

To follow or contact Maja:
Y: www.youtube.com/user/TheAnMish
F: www.facebook.com/majatoudal
T: @majatoudal
To listen or purchase Maja's music:
W: https://majatoudal.bandcamp.com/

Elisabeth Wiklander

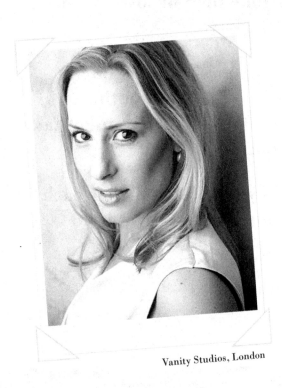

Vanity Studios, London

I am Elisabeth Wiklander from Sweden, aged 33, diagnosed with Asperger Syndrome at age 27

Professional cellist, world-renowned London Philharmonic Orchestra, UK

Previously with the Netherlands Philharmonic in Amsterdam

Master diploma, music. I got my orchestral training in the Royal Concertgebouw Orchestra (Amsterdam), ranked one of the best in the world.

My Strengths:

1. Perseverance and determination

I am a driven person and not afraid to work hard. When I decide to take on a task I always give it all. It does not matter if the task seems impossible or the goal unreachable. I have learned to play a musical instrument and dramatically change some of my behavioural and thinking patterns that were important to change in order to easier co-exist in a mainstream world.

2. Ability to take criticism

Compliments are lovely to receive but to be open to constructive criticism allows me to take in information that gives a more complete picture of myself and how other people perceive me. In my profession it is essential for development. On a personal level, I learn about myself and process the information into useful strategies when it comes to navigating socially.

3. Open mindedness

Learn to be less rigid. Having been strongly opinionated and quite rigid in my thinking, I found myself stuck in patterns and very inflexible when interacting with others. Moving abroad in combination with receiving my diagnosis forced me out of it. Thanks to a lot of practice on changing certain behaviours, learning social skills, looking outside my own sphere, has helped enormously. Furthermore, I have been severely misjudged all my life and watch myself carefully trying not to make the same mistake towards others.

4. Communicating with NTs (neurotypicals are people who are not on the spectrum)

5. Focus when doing something I love/special interest

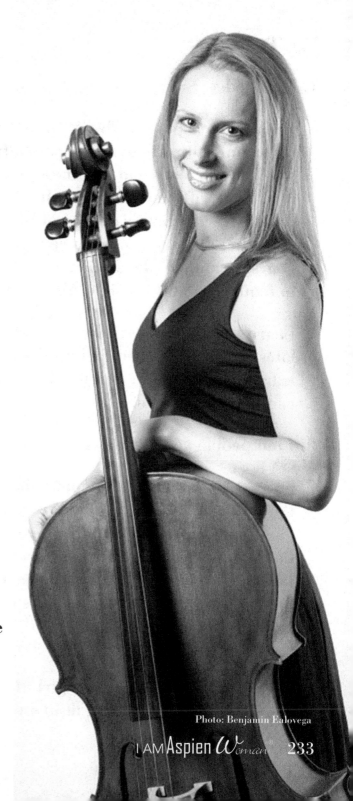

My Top Tips:

1. Knowledge

Knowledge is power. Always strive to learn more about yourself, thereby managing your life more successfully. Challenge yourself and do not be afraid to face your fears and weaknesses. Pain hurts but dealt with in the right way, it will ease off and disappear. It will not kill you and there is great reward on the other side: better quality of life, freedom, peace and strength. Find out why you react the way you do in certain situations, study and learn to understand yourself, almost like a science project. Learn everything you can about Autism in females (and if possible, the most important people around you should too).

Learn what traits you have that relate to Autism and keep up to date with the latest research. Scientific knowledge consistently changes and so do you so keep learning your mind; stay flexible. We can perhaps never become perfect but we can always improve!

2. Find people you can trust

Surround yourself with people who are willing to make an effort to get to know the real you and who will like you for who you are. Do not spend time and energy trying too hard to please others. It might be only one or two friends, family members with whom you are close and of course your spouse if you have one. It is so important to find a partner who is willing to roll up their sleeves to be with you and love you, not in spite of your quirks but because of them.

3. Never quit!

Never, ever give up. I was a girl who was an outsider, alone, strongly disliked people because I couldn't fit in and had a lot of problems until I was diagnosed

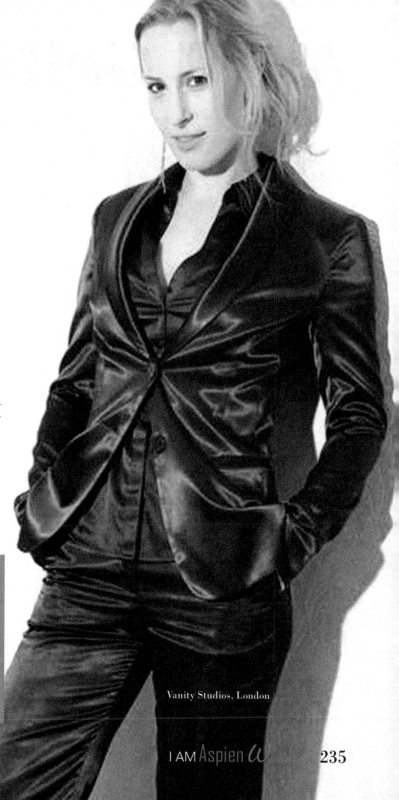

with Asperger's a few years ago. All my youth and childhood I just wanted to hide in the Swedish outback all my life. Now at the age of 33 I live in London, work closely (and successfully) with almost a hundred colleagues and travel internationally to all continents as a member of one of the top orchestras of the world. I managed to establish friendships and be 'part of things', something I wished for all my life but thought I could never have. I worked very hard for it for many years. Today I am in a very happy place.

To follow or contact
Elisabeth:
W: http://www.lpo.org.uk/cello/
elisabeth-wiklander.html
E: elisabeth.wiklander@gmail.com

Vanity Studios, London

April Griffin

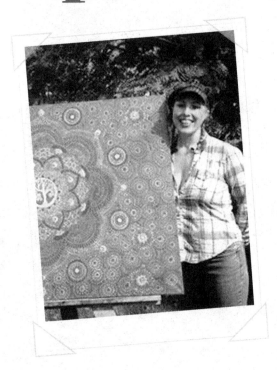

I am April Griffin, aged 39, diagnosed with Autism at age 36

Professional artist, mentor, Autism advocate, environmental activist, Canada

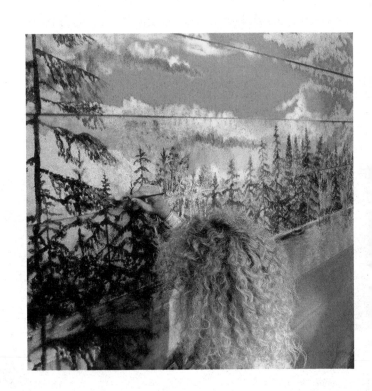

My Strengths:

1. Art, art mentoring and web design

2. Autism advocacy

3. Environmental activism

My Top Tips:

1. Go ahead and be yourself! Find your passion and run with it. Don't worry about what other people think. You have a limited time on earth so the real question is what will you do with it?

2. The best thing I ever did for myself was develop my talents. I started out as an artist at age 8. It led to web design, galleries, photography and now I own my own The Cool Beans Cafe and Gallery and represent other artists too!

3. Find what you love and love who you are!

To contact or follow April:
W: www.facebook.com/aprilgriffinart

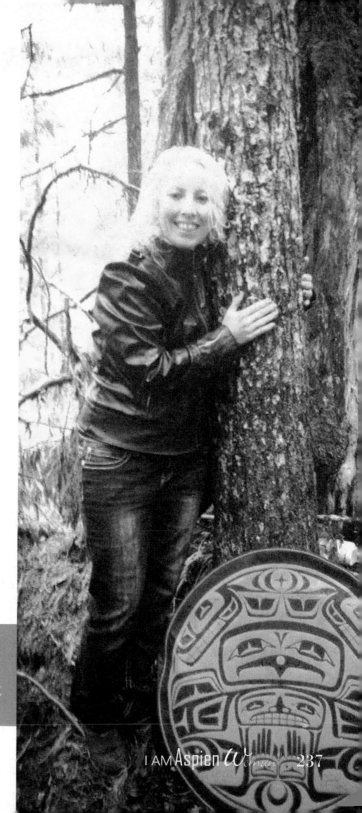

Marguerite (Margo) Comeau

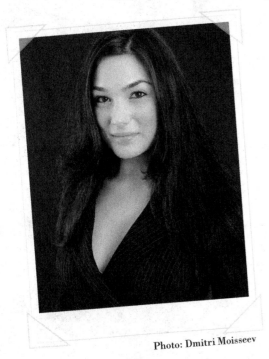

Photo: Dmitri Moisseev

I am Marguerite Comeau, aged 24, diagnosed with Asperger Syndrome at age 23

Author, model, Autism advocate, Canada

My Strengths:

1. Poet, pun artist (writer), blogger and Autism advocate

2. Hyperfocus, exceptional long-term memory

3. Autodidactic (self-taught/directed learner)

4. Model

My Top Tips:

1. Adapt to your surroundings but never change who you are.

2. Learning how to make people laugh goes a long way.

3. Be confident and own your Asperger's; a butterfly is not ashamed that it was once a caterpillar.

Fallen Petals

Believe that roses can grow
from concrete

Only your mask can prevent
you to bloom

Embrace all of you, thorny and
sweet

Fallen petals don't dilute your
perfume

Marguerite Comeau

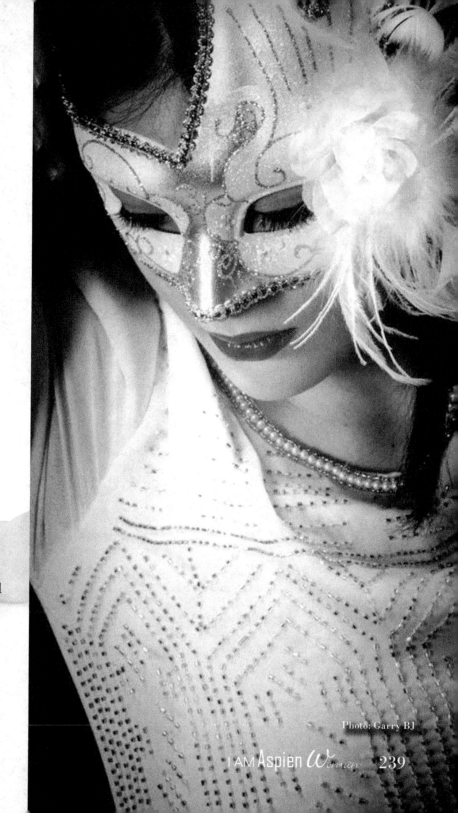

Photo: Garry BJ

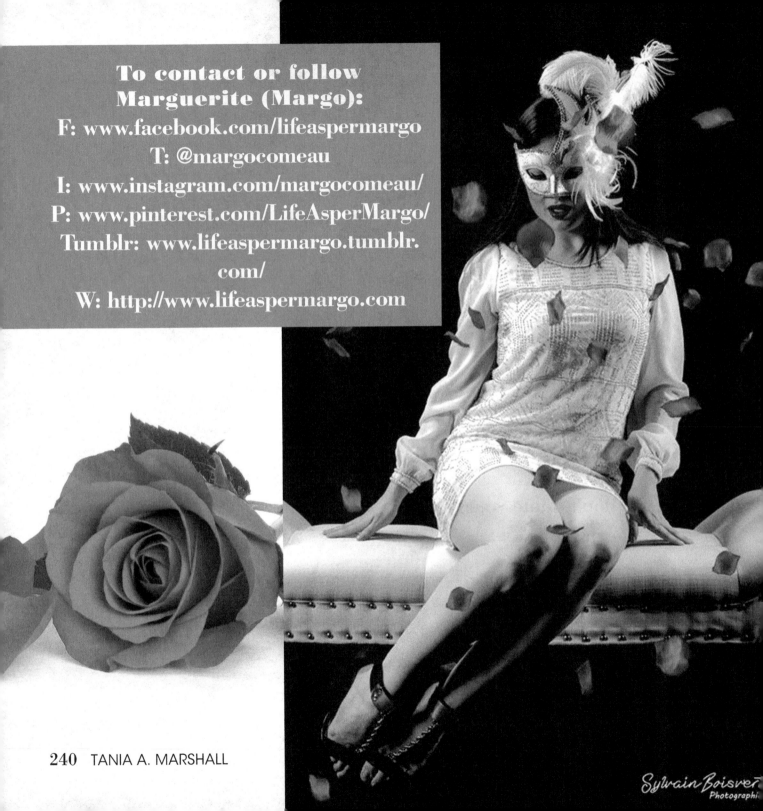

To contact or follow Marguerite (Margo):
F: www.facebook.com/lifeaspermargo
T: @margocomeau
I: www.instagram.com/margocomeau/
P: www.pinterest.com/LifeAsperMargo/
Tumblr: www.lifeaspermargo.tumblr.com/
W: http://www.lifeaspermargo.com

Sylvain Boisvert
Photographi

Annette Harkness

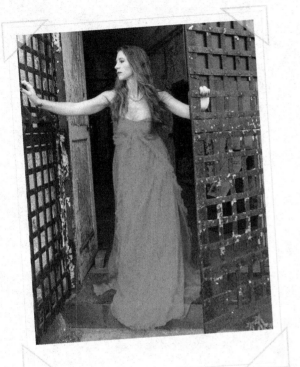

Photo: Laney Lane Photography

I am Annette Harkness, aged 41, diagnosed with Asperger Syndrome at age 35

Professional environmental specialist, a veterinary technician, Autism and interstitial cystitis advocate, model, published writer and poet, photographer, USA

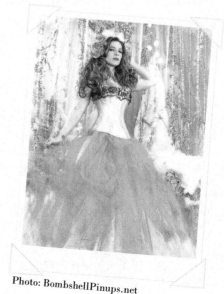

Photo: BombshellPinups.net

My Strengths:

1. Empathetic and compassionate

2. Detail-oriented, gifted and determined

3. Non-judgemental

My Top Tips:

1. Don't ever listen to anyone who tells you that you cannot do something that you want to do.

2. Observe people to learn as much as you can about how neurotypicals interact with each other. This will benefit you greatly, especially when it comes to doing well socially and eventually finding and keeping a good paying job.

3. Be careful in your relationships with people. Sometimes it may be difficult to recognise that you're in a harmful relationship. Educate yourself about harmful personalities.

To contact or follow Annette:
Miss Nettie Fanpages
I: www.instagram.com/
themissnettie
F: www.facebook.com/
missnettiefanpage

DARKNESS

Darkness about me wherever I turn

I reach for a candle

But it does not burn

So much do I long for the light far away

And yet it keeps moving

Further each day

I follow behind

A hint of hope in my eyes

Desperately trying to capture the light

I am drawn to the light

As a moth in the night

And so it is said

Darkness craves light

Annette Stanton-Harkness

Megan Barnes

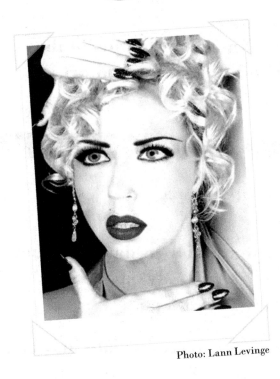

Photo: Lann Levinge

I am Megan Barnes, aged 34, diagnosed with Asperger Syndrome at age 30

I am a professional singer and actress, Australia

My Strengths:

1. Acute powers of observation, unique ability to mimic celebrities; I sing, choreograph, costume design, dance, act in caricature, produce alongside Lann Levinge (Levinge Events) in Lady Gaga, P!nk, Katy Perry, Madonna and Ke$ha tribute shows. One of my favourite gigs is performing for the disabled and Down syndrome people.

2. Quality and attention to detail, amazing business ideas

3. Learning and storing constant new material and performing in front of (sometimes) thousands of people. I've honed these skills because of focus, perseverance and determination

4. Visually sensitive to coordinating colours and knowing what fits in the sense, having a flair for interior decorating and Photoshop and art

My Top Tips:

1. There are still people who won't understand you in day-to-day life. They may try to change you to do or act as they see is best. My advice is: it's ok to try new ways of doing things and actively give it a go.

2. One of the super powers gained from learning my diagnosis late in life. I learned much patience, tolerance and acceptance for ANY person different or the same as I. I wanted to treat others the way I wished to be treated.

3. As a singer it is my job to keep as many people happy at the same time as possible. And at times that has required new ideas. For things to grow sometimes they must change.

4. Believe in yourself and your strengths will shine. With my singing, I have always performed my best using my own 'knowing'.

5. Learn what brings you calm/peace and know that it's a good thing to make time for every day. To recharge your batteries and know that whatever you face in your day you still have that to come back to.

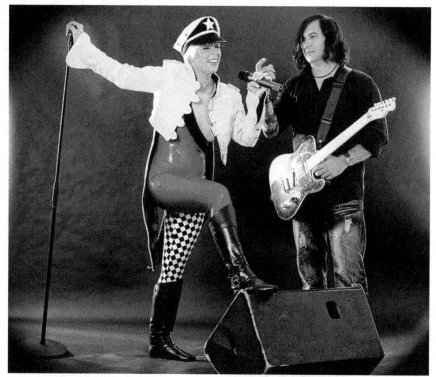

PINK Tribute Show | Photo: IsaacInsoll.com

To contact or follow Megan:
W: www.zookeepers.com.au/
W: www.levinge.com.au/
T: @MeganBarnes
Pink Tribute Show
https://www.facebook.com/PinksTributeShow?pnref=lhc
Katy Perry Tribute Show
https://www.facebook.com/KatyPerryTribute?pnref=lhc
Lady Gaga Tribute Show
https://www.facebook.com/ladygagatribute?pnref=lhc

Samantha Craft

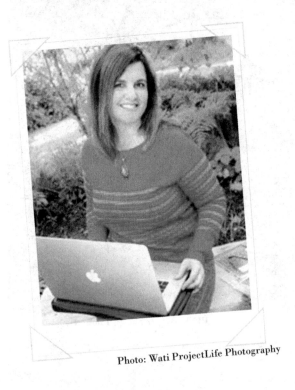

Photo: Wati ProjectLife Photography

I am Samantha Craft, aged 46, diagnosed with Asperger Syndrome at age 44

Writer, educator and Autism advocate, USA

My Strengths:

1. Artistic ability

2. Writing and blogging

3. Helping others and educating

My Top Tips:

1. Immerse yourself in your creative passions. Create from the inner you born in beauty. Share your gifts and talents with others. Share your story, your truth and your heart.

2. Expose yourself to people who resonate at a high-vibration of acceptance. Break up with all relations that feed off your energy, goodness, innocence, and purity. Establish an environment in which you can be your authentic, shining self.

3. Understand you need no fixing or alterations. Concentrate on the manmade definitions of 'imperfection', 'flawed', 'wrong' and 'normal', and realise their limitations. Learn everything you can about the Autistic spectrum through reputable, well-honoured sources. Look into healthy personal blog accounts, websites, local groups and social network support groups online. And then forget all that you have learned and recognise you are a unique individual with exact perfection.

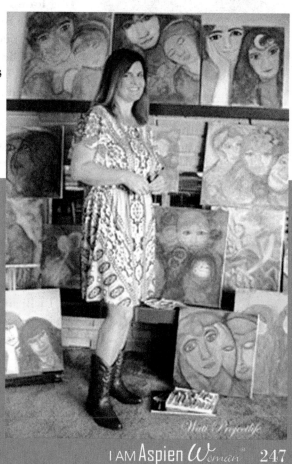

To contact or follow Sam:
Blog: aspergersgirls.wordpress.com
Find a community on Facebook at 'Samantha Craft' at Everyday Asperger's
F: www.facebook.com/pages/Everyday-Aspergers/387026824645012?__mref=message_bubble
Watch for *Full Circle*, by Samantha Craft, a support book for females on the spectrum, coming soon.

Genevieve Kingston

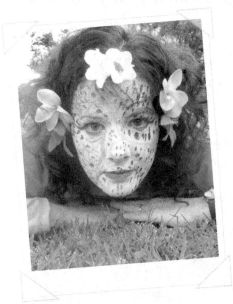

I am Genevieve Kingston, aged 43, self-diagnosed with Asperger Syndrome at age 41

Wife, mother, registered midwife, Australia.

My Top Tips:

1   I found out three years ago that I have Asperger's. It was a huge relief because now I understood why I have always been perceived as weird. Finding out I have Asperger's allowed me to be kinder to myself.

2   I have found my strengths and I use them. Finding out what your strengths and weaknesses are, and allowing those to just be, will go a long way to you being at peace with yourself.

3.   I don't listen to the news; I have enough heartbreak at work, I don't need the misery on the news. I will sit and sob for hours after some news reports and I am gentle towards myself when I've put my foot in it.

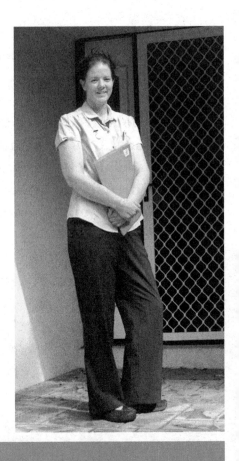

My Strengths:

1. I'm exceptionally good at reading people

2. I take care of my empathic side

3. Midwifery

Genevieve is on Twitter at
T: @ladybirdsrred

248   TANIA A. MARSHALL

Brandy Nightingale

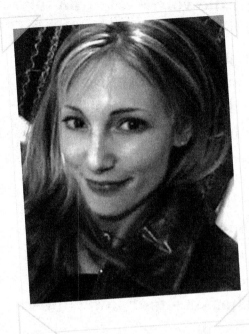

I am Brandy Nightingale, aged 39, diagnosed with Autism at age 35

USA

My Strengths:

1. Visual effects co-ordinator

2. Own my own pet care business (www.thepeacefulpup.com)

3. Retired stand-up comedian (performed for eight years)

4. Survivor of childhood physical, mental, emotional and sexual abuse. I'm a survivor of school bullying

5. Active blogger (http://brandynightingale.blogspot.com)

6. The *RebelSpark Project* is an online video series introducing youth to adults who have carved unique paths for themselves despite challenges, differences and disabilities. Check for updates on twitter: @RebelSparkTV

My Top Tips:

1. My take away from life and the wisdom I'd like to pass along to fellow female Aspiens is this: listen to yourself without the voices and opinions of others. Really sit with yourself and listen to what your body tells you about your needs, wants, and most of all, your passions and talents. What makes you feel giddy inside? What can you spend hours working on? What is it you do that seems to make time disappear? If your body wants to read, by all means let it read. If your body wants to write, by all means write! If your body wants to build, by all means let it build!

2. Although we all have responsibilities such as school, work, or even families to care for, we MUST make time for our passions and develop our talents. We Aspiens are more specialists than generalists, meaning we can be really good or even genius at a topic or two, beyond what most can comprehend. Isn't that incredible? That's a superpower most of us share. It is people like us who create new gadgets, who have a special ability to connect with animals, who have a special ability to focus on small details of tasks for much longer than others. We are the ones who have the innate ability to solve problems for the world. More than ever, the world needs our superpowers, so let's fine-tune them and let them shine!

To contact or follow Brandy:
Everything's Hunky Dory
Blog: brandynightingale.blogspot.com
F: www.facebook.com/everythingshunkydory

Shan Ellis Williams

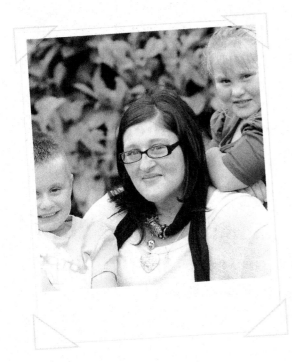

I am Shân Ellis Williams, aged 37, diagnosed with Asperger Syndrome in 2014 on the day of my 37th birthday

I am an editor and a columnist with two UK national papers, mother of two (one of them is also on the spectrum) and I run ASDigest magazine in my spare time

My Strengths:

1. Optimism

2. Openness and understanding

3. Writer and editor

To contact or follow Shan:
F: facebook.com/blodyntatws
T: @awdures
Skype: Shan.ellis1

My Top Tips:

1. Always to follow your heart.

2. Don't be undermined by people who tell you can't do something. You can. You have the power to do whatever you want, however you want, and if you have a goal in mind, always reach towards it.

Sybelle Silverphoenix

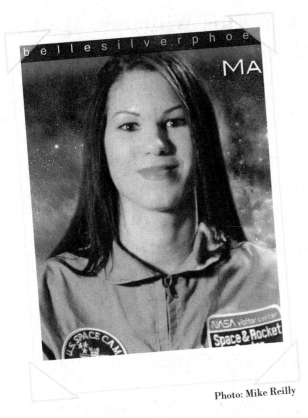

Photo: Mike Reilly

I am Sybelle Silverphoenix, aged 31, diagnosed with Asperger Syndrome at age 27

MarsOne Round 2 Finalist 2013 selection, actress, model and singer, New York, USA

My Strengths:

1. Fixing computers

2. MarsOne project applicant, waiting for my one-way ticket to Mars. In July 2013, I applied for the Mars One space mission to colonise the red planet. Over 200,000 applications were received, and the initial

set of applicants to make round two were 1,058. After round two medical examinations, that number was reduced to 663 globally. We then were candidates awaiting interviews to determine passage into round three of the program, which is slated to be televised through Darlow Smithson Productions (responsible for such programs as Stephen Hawking's Universe and Grand Design)

3. Former lead vocalist for the rock band Kings Valentine

4. Self-taught portrait sketcher, quick learner, Autism advocate

5. Actress, director, model and dancer

My Top Tips:

1. People will try to put you in the proverbial box you won't fit into, not just for being on the Spectrum, but also because you are female. In a world full of double standards for women, you must defy because you are not a stereotype of what a woman must 'be', you are creating a world where we are judged less by stereotypes and more by our own merit.

2. Create your own environment so you can be yourself. Start your own business, for example, so you have no one else to answer to.

3. Be fearless. Love who you are because there are no duplicates and that is more valuable than being a conformist, despite how others may treat you.

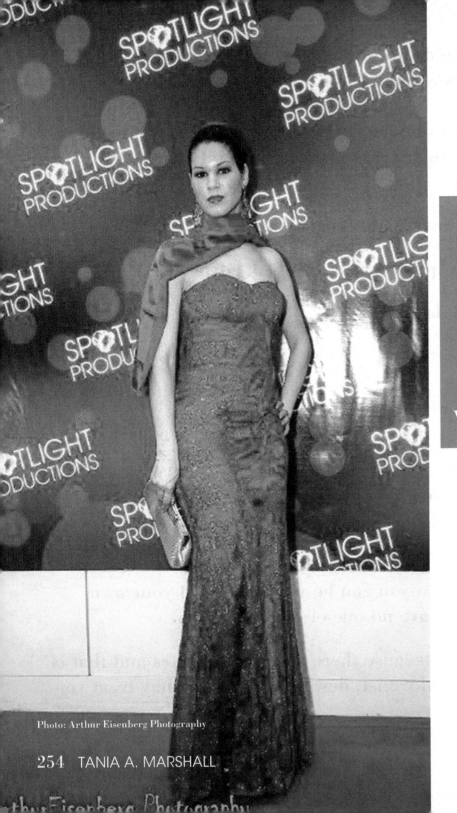

Photo: Arthur Eisenberg Photography

254 TANIA A. MARSHALL

To contact or follow Sybelle:
T: @SybelleSilver
F: facebook.com/Sybelle Silverphoenix
I: SybelleSilverphoenix
Ello: Sybelle_Silverphoenix
W: sybellesilverphoenix.com

Dena Gassner

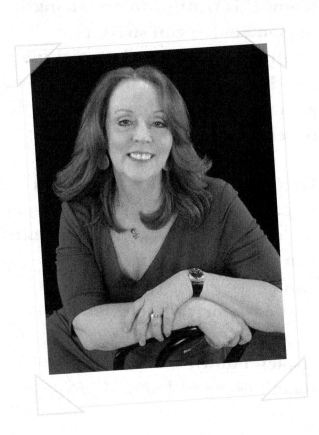

I am Dena Gassner, aged 56, diagnosed with Autism at age 38

I am a master's degree social worker, working on my PhD in social welfare

I am a wife, mother and grandmother, USA

My list of strengths:

1. Perseverance

2. Dedication

3. Writing

4. The passion to leave a legacy of change

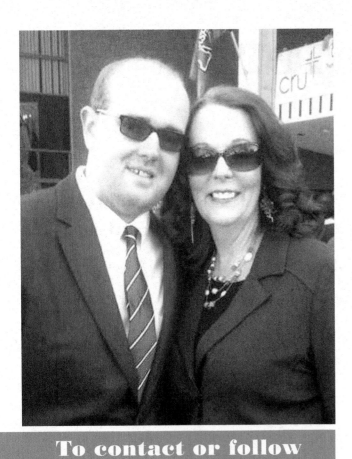

To contact or follow Dena:

Dena Gassner. LMSW – Program Director, Center for Understanding

W: www.denagassner.com/

E: c4ucontact@gmail.com

F: www.facebook.com/pages/Center-For-Understanding/211788052343

My Top Tips:

1. Know this truth: you are enough. AspienWomen can strive to be superwomen rather than seeking to be whatever personal best they can achieve. Aim for that and you will never fail!

2. Care for yourself first, above all else. If you are unhappy or unsafe in your home, work or community, you are slowly killing yourself. You can't care for anyone until you first care for yourself. Part of this is being 'in community' with your Aspien family. Don't stay in the loneliness of isolation. Find your people!

3. Do what you love and you will love what you do. Find a way to pursue your gifts ideally, first as a career, but at least as a hobby because these gifts are your joy and happiness.

Xolie Morra Cogley of Xolie Morra & The Strange Kind

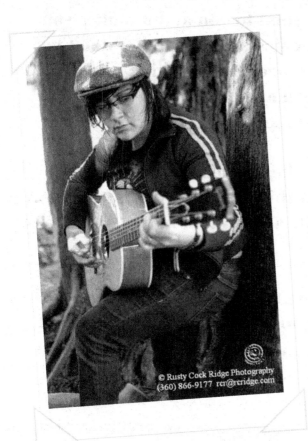

© Rusty Cock Ridge Photography
(360) 866-9177 rcr@rcridge.com

I am Xolie Morra Cogley, age 35 and diagnosed with Autism at age 31

I am a singer, songwriter and producer, USA

My list of strengths:

1. Perfect pitch

2. Thinking in music/sound

3. Mimicking noises really well

As a songwriter, I hear songs fully produced the first time it pops into my mind. I also hear other people's songs fully produced the first time I hear them. I can also hear when someone is a fraction of a hair off from the proper note and don't even get me started on the sound created by automated tuning programs!

My Top Tips:

1. The most important advice I can give to any human on the spectrum, female, male or intersex, is to only strive to be 'Your Normal'. If your normal is putting on an accent that sounds good to you and it makes you feel good and stops your stuttering or motor tics, then do it, but don't try to talk or act like 'The Cool Kid' clique just because you think it will make you fit in with them. You be you, because you are cooler than any cool kid could ever dream of being, because you see the world in a very cool way.

2. Study and learn sarcasm. Learning about these things has helped me make better decisions about how I react to things that I might otherwise have taken very literally. While you're at it, add human body language to the list of things to study.

3. Talk about your Autism openly. It's nothing to be ashamed of. Most of my social issues came from not being diagnosed. I fit in by pretending I knew what was going on. Being diagnosed and then opening up about that diagnosis helped break down the wall that people put up.

To contact or follow Xolie:
W: http://www.thestrangekind.com
T: @TheStrangeKind
F: www.facebook.com/TheStrangeKind

Photo: Rusty Cock Ridge Photography

Jessica Ivey

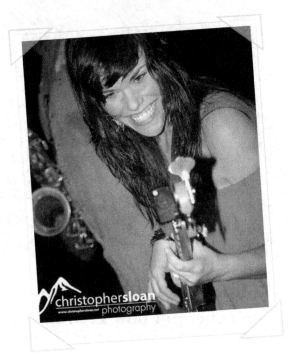

I am Jessica Ivey, aged 35 and diagnosed at age 34, USA

'Mum' to a wonderful son (Kevin), bassist and artist at JiveyStarStudios, practice manager at a medical centre

Currently enrolled in a master's to PhD (bridge program) for clinical pastoral counselling.

My Strengths:

1. Keen Aspie instinct

2. Intense dedication

3. Musician

4. Artist

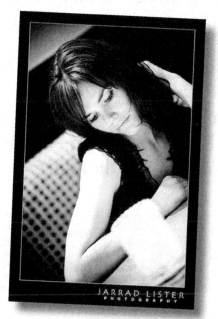

My Top Tips:

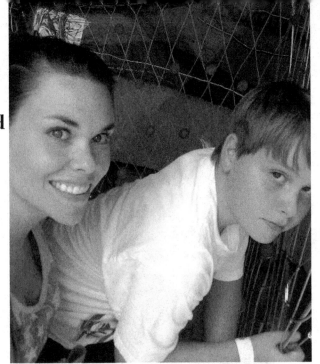

1. Do not to be afraid to seek out a formal diagnosis. A paradigm shift has occurred in my life since that day. Identifying myself with others 'like' me has given form to my many faces and what I found in the centre was not another mask, but my validated identity. A diagnosis at any age gives you an understanding of why things have been difficult if they have been, and a stepping stone towards moving forward into the future.

2. Learn what works for best for sensory-related obstacles. I struggle with clothes 'pulling' on me. I have adjusted my wardrobe and now getting ready in the morning is a little easier.

3. Use executive function apps. Set a countdown on your phone where you can see it, instead of an alarm or reminder. This really helps me complete tasks and not become fixated with the shift. I also keep a couple of 'Bright Ideas' lists on neon paper around my house. That way I can jot down things as soon as they surface in my mind.

To contact or follow Jessica:
P: www.pinterest.com/JIveyStarStudio

Lexington Sherbin

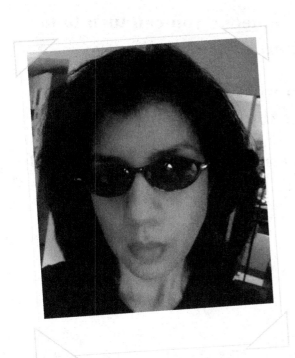

I am Lexington Sherbin, aged 41 and diagnosed with Autism at age 41

Los Angeles, California, USA

Professional writer/screenwriter/artist and singer (tenor)

My Strengths:

1. Writing

2. Painting

3. Singing

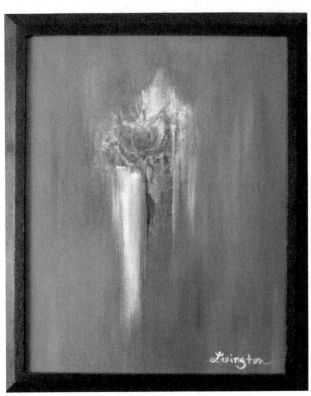

Art by Lexington Sherbin

My Top Tips:

1. Have someone you can turn to for help and advice.

2. Learn what helps you and what makes things harder for you.

3. Forget about comparing yourself to others. Be your special, unique self!

Lexington can be contacted or followed at:
Artwork can be viewed on artla.com here:
W: http://art.exelsites.com/artists/artist.cfm?m=396

YouTube video: Irlen and Sensory Perception and Light Sensitivity ASD
Y: https://www.youtube.com/watch?v=MVpbdGFeEqI

APPENDIX 1
Commonly observed characteristics, traits and strengths of adult females

Some Commonly Observed Characteristics, Traits and Strengths of Adult Females

Disclaimer: This is not a diagnostic test. Please take this detailed list to a professional who preferably has some knowledge of/or specialises in female Autism/Asperger Syndrome, if you or someone you know identifies with the majority of traits. This table is based on clinic experiences, observations, anecdotal evidence, and descriptions by other women with Autism or Asperger Syndrome. There is a great need for female-based research. Autism tends to be a *condition of extremes*; for example females tend to be either superior with or disabled by mathematics. It is also important to remember that Autism is a heterogeneous condition, and therefore, no two females with Autism will be the same or experience the same characteristics or to the same degree.

This list typifies many of the AspienWomen I have worked with. These traits also depend to some extent on the severity, whether you've been assessed and diagnosed and/or received support and intervention, and also whether there is additional co-existing condition(s) (e.g. a personality disorder) present.

1. Cognitive/intellectual abilities

Tend to have high average to genius intelligence, may have significant splits between verbal and perceptual reasoning abilities, lower working memory and/or processing speeds, learning disabilities (e.g. dyscalculia, dyslexia, reading comprehension).

Superior long-term memory.

Weaker short-term memory.

Usually need academic accommodations in university.

An uneven profile of abilities; a distinct profile consisting of strengths and weaknesses, learning disabilities/ differences.

May experience rigid negative thinking, inflexible black or white thinking style.

Specialist thinkers, often good at one thing and not so good at other things with each of the three types of thinking on a continuum.

A. Word/fact thinkers
This type of thinker prefers words and speech and has a great memory for a variety of facts. Verbal specialists who are good at talking and writing but usually lack visual skills.

B. Visual thinkers
Visual thinkers think and 'see' in images or moving pictures. They need to 'see' things in order to learn and/or understand them. They are often artists or photographers. Visual thinkers are often poor at algebra.

C. Pattern thinkers
Patterns thinkers find patterns in everything. They tend to be excellent at music or mathematics, and may have problems with reading or writing composition.

1. Cognitive/intellectual abilities

Executive functioning difficulties may include: trouble making decisions, time management, planning ahead, organisation, completing tasks.

Photographic visual memory.

2. Education/university life

May have dropped out of high school and gone back later, or may have repeated a grade. May have unfinished or partial degrees, may have many finished degrees, many have PhD level qualifications. Many have taken longer to achieve their education, as compared to their peers.

May have a history of enrolling and attending university classes, followed by dropping out of classes or semesters. She then re-enrols/attends later on in life. This is usually due to being overloaded and overwhelmed. A history of deferring exams, not attending classes, dropping out of classes or programs is common.

May have repeated high school or courses OR dropped out completely.

A history of many doctor and counsellor visits throughout university life, without any significant improvement.

Difficulty taking the same amount of courses or classes as her peers.

May get lost on campus easily, lose possessions, be late for classes or exams.

3. Career/work

Often drawn to the helping, artistic or animal professions, and often an 'expert' in her chosen field. I know of many AspienWomen who are successful in the following careers: artists, singers, actors, poets, writers, teachers, psychologists, psychiatrists, special needs teachers/consultants, horse trainers/whisperers, doctors, scientists, accountants, authors, childcare workers, models, comedians, artists, computer-related specialists, animal handlers or zoo keepers, university professors, nurses, medical intuitives, entrepreneurs and photographers.

May miss days of work due to social exhaustion.

May find great difficulty attending/participating in staff meetings, lunch breaks, work social events.

May make up excuses for not attending work/staff functions.

May have a history of being unable to cope with work/employment environments, often moving from job to job, especially in younger adult years.

Hard-working, conscientious worker.

May get stressed if have a lot of work to do in a short amount of time.

May become frustrated/stressed if asked to do too many things at once.

Tries very hard to avoid making mistakes, forgetting things.

www.aspiengirl.com © Tania A. Marshall

3. Career/work

Tries hard to please others.

May burn bridges (e.g. walk out or quit jobs or relationships without notice).

4. Social and friendships/relationships

Preference for one-on-one social interactions, single close friendships.

May flitter and have many acquaintances or know many people but no deep relationships with them.

Need more time away from people than their peers (solitude).

May experience stress, anxiety and confusion in social group or group work situations.

Strong preference to engage in conversation related to their special interest.

Strong dislike for social chit-chat, gossip, nonsense, lies or conversation that lacks a 'function' to it, but some are known to engage in it themselves.

A history of being bullied, teased, left out and/or not fitting in with same-age peers, unless she had/has similar 'Aspie' friends.

An intense dislike of lies, but may lie herself.

Has an ability to socialise; however, is unable to do so for long periods of time. Suffers from 'social exhaustion' or a 'social hangover' when socialising too much. The hangover can last hours to days, which can be debilitating.

Experience great difficulty with conflict, arguments, being yelled at, fighting, war.

Has great difficulty asserting herself, asking for help, setting boundaries.

May need to drink to be able to socialise.

May currently have or have experienced post-traumatic stress, often due to being misunderstood, misdiagnosed, mistreated, and/or mis-medicated.

Social skills differences – is exceptionally good one-on-one and presenting to groups; however, has difficulty working within group situations.

May find herself in social situations or relationships that she is unhappy with, but not know how to remove herself from them.

History of being taken advantage of by others, even though she has taken the appropriate business, legal or social advice from others.

Often bored in social situations or parties and/or does not know how to act in social situations.

May say 'yes' to social events, then later make up an excuse as to why she cannot attend, often staying home in solitude (reading a book or engaging in her special interest).

Often prefers to be engaged in her special interest, rather than socialising.

4. Social and friendships/relationships

May be considered the 'black sheep' of the family.

Others consider her different, odd, eccentric or 'weird'.

May feel like she has to act 'normal' to please others OR does not care at all about fitting in.

Copies, mimics, acts in order to fit in and make others like her.

A people pleaser, but then may burn bridges suddenly (e.g. quit relationships), as they have difficulty managing conflict.

Females appear to be better than males at masking the traits of Autism in social situations. However, girls are less able to do so in unfamiliar settings.

May be considered a 'loner' OR may have many acquaintances, but no real friends.

May have an intense desire to please others and/ be liked by others. May become highly distressed if she has the perception that someone does not like her or actually does not like her.

May have spent a lifetime of using enormous effort to socially 'pretend', 'fake it', 'fit in', 'pass for normal'. May have utilised body language books, mirrors, acting/drama classes to improve social skills.

5. Communication

Difficulties communicating her thoughts and feelings, in words, to others, especially if anxious, stressed or upset. Often can type or write her thoughts much better.

There may be a tendency towards the following:

Dislikes asking others for help, be unable to ask or not know how to ask for help.

Displays passivity, not know how to assert her boundaries in a healthy manner.

Offends others by saying what she is thinking, even if she does not mean to.

Points out other people's mistakes.

Gives too much detail and end up boring others unintentionally.

Asks embarrassing questions (usually when younger).

Unusual voice (flat, monotone, high-pitched, child-like).

Tendency to take things literally, missing what people are trying to say.

May talk too loudly or too softly; often unaware that she is doing so.

Often surprised when people tell her she has been rude or inappropriate.

Poor pragmatic language skills; the social use of language.

May regress to the use of an immature social skills set when stressed.

A. Highly sensitive

High sensitivity, may not be able to listen to or watch the news, listen to the radio, read the newspaper, watch violent shows/movies or horror movies, see hurt or injured animals, abuse, war, trauma, are sensitive to the emotions and 'emotional atmosphere' of the environment, experience referred emotion and strong intuitive 'sixth sense' abilities or mirror-touch synesthesia (needs more research, see resources section).

B. Sensory processing disorder/condition

May have sensory sensitivities in the following areas: hearing, vision, taste, touch, smell, balance, movement, intuition, will either seek or avoid stimulation in each area.

May have synesthesia.

May be very sensitive to pain or have a high pain threshold.

May notice how food tastes or feels and one may be more important than the other.

May be clumsy or un-coordinated.

May dislike loud noises and/or be overwhelmed or stressed by bright lights, strong smells, coarse textures/clothing, sirens close by or people too close behind her.

May find children hard to cope with due to crying, screaming or other loud noises.

Sensitive to the way clothes feel and how they may be more important than how they look.

May have to withdraw, isolate herself when overwhelmed by her senses.

May not be able to tolerate sounds, sights, smells, textures, movement that she dislikes.

May not like to be hugged, cuddled or held. "I only like to hug if it's my decision".

May either love sensual or sexual touch or dislike it intensely.

Can get upset or distressed if unable to follow a familiar route when going somewhere.

Things that should feel painful may not be (bruises but not know how they got there, due to clumsiness).

In social situations, the nervous system tends to be overwhelmed easily, leading to withdrawal (e.g. wander off to a quiet spot at a party, play with children or animals).

Strong hunger may disrupt her mood and/or ability to focus.

She may notice and enjoy delicate or fine scents, tastes, sounds, works of art and pieces of music.

Often does certain things with hands (twirling hair or items, different movements) or legs (leg 'bouncing' or rocking while standing) or rubbing feet together.

www.aspiengirl.com © Tania A. Marshall

7. Physical Appearance

Usually dresses differently from her peers, often eccentric, may dress more for comfort than appearance.

May dress 'over the top' or unusually for occasions, may love makeup, clothes and fashion, may be a trend-setter.

May try very hard to fit in appearance wise or may not care at all. Some spend inordinate amounts of time with grooming, makeup and clothing, and organising outfits.

May not shower or upkeep hygiene at times, due to different priorities (usually being involved in special interests).

A tendency to look and act younger than her years.

8. Lifestyle

Books, computers, the Internet, animals, children, nature may be her best friends.

She loves quiet, solitude, peaceful surroundings.

She may be ultra-religious or not at all. Buddhism appears to be common.

May prefer to spend as much time as possible by herself, with animals or in nature.

May have a strong preference for routine and things being the same day after day.

Gets pleasure from being engaged in her chosen work and/or special interests rather than socialising.

9. Relationship choices/sexuality/gender

May date or marry much older or much younger partners, same gender partner, tending not to see the 'age' or 'gender', but rather the personality of the person first.

May be asexual, having preferences that are deemed as more important than sex or a relationship.

May be 'hypersexual', fascinated by physical sexual contact.

May differ from peers in terms of flexibility regarding sexual orientation or may think about or want to change gender. Some individuals may change gender or experiment with sexuality as a means to find social success or to 'fit in' or feel less different.

May not have wanted or needed intimate relationships (asexual).

There is a greater flexibility in sexuality and/or gender. May be heterosexual or may be asexual, gay, lesbian, bisexual or transgender.

May have gender dysphoria, also known as gender identity disorder (GID) dysphoria, and is a formal diagnosis for individuals who feel and experience significant stress and unhappiness with their birth gender and/or gender roles. These individuals are known as transsexual or transgender.

www.aspiengirl.com © Tania A. Marshall

10. Special Interests

A special interest may involve the person's career, feminism, justice studies, law, philosophy, psychology, the field of self-help, neuroscience, English literature, language, fantasy, teaching, education and special needs, Autism, writing, art, music, fashion and makeup, animals, lifelong learning, celebrities, tattoos and symbols.

Ability to 'hyperfocus' for long periods of time involved in the special interest, without eating, drinking or going to the toilet, is able to hyperfocus on her special interest for hours, often losing track of time.

Loves and revels in solitude, peace and quiet. Solitude is often described as 'needing it like the air I breathe'.

An intense love for nature and animals.

Often not interested in what other people find interesting.

May collect or hoard items of interest.

May make it a high priority to arrange her life, events, work and environment to avoid overwhelming, stressful or upsetting situations.

11. Emotional

Feels things deeply.

Other people's moods affect her, especially if they are negative.

Tends to be very sensitive to emotional pain.

Deeply moved by arts, music, certain movies.

May be unable to watch horror, violence, disturbing movies and news programs.

Lives with continual generalised anxiety, bouts of depression that creep up on her.

Difficulty regulating emotions and managing stress.

Is socially and emotionally younger/more immature than her chronological age, much younger if in her twenties.

Emotionally too honest (inability or difficulty hiding true feelings when it would be more socially acceptable to do so) and naive.

Experiences intense emotions of all kinds (e.g. when she falls in love, she 'falls' in love deeply).

May think she is being compassionate, but her actions may not come across that way.

Often too sensitive and possesses a lot of empathy.

Usually connects and/or are very sensitive to certain characters in movies.

Highly sensitive to issues affecting earth, animals, people, advocacy, justice, human rights and the 'underdog'.

Some women are quite 'child-like', not reaching a maturity until roughly 40 years of age.

12. Personality characteristics and/or traits and abilities

May be characterised by a subtype, e.g. tomboy, fashion diva, domestic diva, academic, actress, bookworm, athlete.

Intelligent.

Usually has more than one gift.

A natural born leader, independent, strong-willed, determined and can be highly competitive (even with herself).

High levels of introversion OR can be extraverted.

Generally lack a strong sense of self, self-esteem and/or identity. May use chameleon-like skills to assimilate and be involved with to a variety of groups or different people over time, in a search for true identity.

Has a high sense of justice and fairness, is a truth-seeker, may have a misguided sense of justice.

Highly creative and may have 'rushes' of original ideas.

Dislikes change and may find it disorienting and stressful.

Highly sensitive to criticism or perceived criticism.

Dislikes being observed when having to perform (performance anxiety).

May have been told she cares too much, does too much for others and/or is too sensitive.

Is perfectionistic (may have attended a perfectionism group program).

Attention to detail.

Obsessions/special interests can be short term (switching from one to another quickly) or long term (can make a great career).

Naivety, innocence, trusting too much and taking others literally are a powerful concoction for being misused and abused.

A strong sense of feeling different from her peers, often described as being from a different planet.

May not have a sense of self and/or identity, self-esteem.

Tend to be very serious, often too serious at times.

Is intense in everything she does.

In childhood, may have been described as highly sensitive and/or shy.

An intense and continual need to figure oneself out.

13. Past and/or current mental health history

May have a history of crying a lot, without knowing why.

Usually a lengthy history of going to therapists, psychiatrists, psychologists.

May have tried a variety of medications.

13. Past and/or current mental health history

Experiences social anxiety and generalised anxiety disorder.

May have Obsessive Compulsive Disorder or traits.

May have one or more of the seven types of ADHD.

Has experienced ongoing depression and/or tiredness/exhaustion, without knowing why.

A history of trying to understand oneself, of finding answers to explain one-self and why she feels she is different or doesn't fit in, as a woman.

A history of many doctor and counsellor visits throughout university life.

May have a family history of Autism, Asperger Syndrome, bipolar disorder, schizophrenia, ADHD, OCD, anxiety disorders, alcoholism.

May have been misdiagnosed with bipolar disorder, borderline personality disorder or schizophrenia, schizoaffective disorder.

May have been diagnosed with anxiety disorder depression, an eating disorder, borderline personality disorder, bipolar disorder and/or ADHD.

A history of depression, anxiety, eating issues or an eating disorder, mood swings.

May have particular phobias (e.g. tocophobia, a fear of childbirth or fear of death starting in childhood).

14. Coping Mechanisms

May have turned to alcohol, drugs, smoking in order to cope with intense emotions, self-medicate and/or socialise/ fit in and/or be accepted within a group.

May use a different persona when out in the public, in order to cope.

May use exercise and have exercise addiction, becoming injured due to too much training.

Gives the impression she is an athlete, may train as if she is training for a marathon but when you ask her she says she isn't training for anything in particular.

May have developed a variety of dysfunctional coping mechanisms (e.g. arrogance and/or narcissism).

May change gender or sexuality in an attempt to 'fit it' and/or find the right group.

Has used imitation, social echolalia, to pretend to be normal, fake it or pass for normal.

May sway from side to side or rock standing up, lying down, in a rocking chair to calm down or self-soothe.

May need to withdraw into bed or a dark area or a place of solitude to gain privacy, quiet and manage sensory and/ or social overload.

Withdrawal and/or avoidance.

May have developed a personality disorder as a means of coping with Asperger Syndrome.

14. Coping Mechanisms

May have developed an eating disorder.

15. Intuitive abilities

Has the ability to feel other people's emotions.

May 'know' or have knowledge of certain things, but no idea how she knows.

May use abilities in a professional capacity, i.e. medical intuitive.

Possesses one or more intuitive abilities.

Is an 'empath'.

Identifies with being a highly sensitive person (HSP).

16. Some common unique abilities and strengths

Intelligence, craves knowledge and loves learning.

Can teach herself just about anything she puts her mind to.

Has a strong will, is determined and independent.

Perfectionistic.

Have a remarkable long-term memory, photographic memory.

A great sense of humour.

Can work very well in a 'crisis' situation, but may fall apart afterwards.

Deeply reflective thinker.

Resilience, an ability to go from one crisis to another, to bounce back, to start again time and time again.

Attention to detail.

Great in one-on-one situations or presenting to a group.

More like 'philosophers' than 'professors', but can be both.

Seeing in the 'mind's eye' exact details, gifted visual learner.

May be gifted with art, music, writing, languages.

Highly intuitive.

Capable of deep philosophical thinking, females with Asperger's often become writers, poets, artists, singers, performers, actresses or professors.

www.aspiengirl.com © Tania A. Marshall

17. Challenges

May be difficult to understand subtle emotions, e.g. when someone is jealous or embarrassed, uninterested or bored.

Often misperceives and misinterprets other's intentions.

A tendency to 'shoot first' and ask questions later.

An 'enlarged justice gland' can be a positive or a negative. The challenge for some individuals is a stubborn viewpoint coupled with inflexibility, a lack of compromise and/or being 'hyper-principled'. Some individuals continue to hold their view (which is perceived to be right), despite obvious personal, negative and/or destructive personal cost to them or themselves.

Keeping up appearances, passing for normal.

May be too 'militant' in their 'causes', lacking the social tact required to gain followers.

Managing emotions.

Learning difficulties.

Rigid thinking, negative thinking.

May get very upset with unexpected change.

May not be able to tell when someone is flirting with her.

Challenging to work and function within a group.

Great difficulty and very sensitive to conflict, stress, arguments, fighting, wars, gossip and negativity. May believe the gossip they hear due to social naivety.

Social chit-chat, small talk, conversation without a 'function', maintaining friendships and relationships, social anxiety or social phobia.

May like or prefer to be by herself as much as possible.

May find it challenging to understand what others expect of her.

Being taken advantage of due to naivety, innocence and trusting others too much.

Boundary issues.

May have difficulty filling out forms, doing paperwork (completing taxes), budgeting money.

May have difficulty recognising or remembering faces (prosopagnosia).

May have Borderline Personality Disorder traits or meet criteria for Borderline Personality Disorder, making the diagnostic picture and treatment more complex.

May also have a personality disorder, in addition to Autism.

Often regresses to child-like behaviours/responses when stressed, anxious or angry.

Theory of mind and context blindness issues.

18. Empathy

May have a lack of cognitive empathy and hyper-empathy (e.g. too much affective empathy).

Cognitive empathy: The ability to predict other's thoughts and intentions, knowing how the other person feels and what they might be thinking. Also known as perspective-taking.

Affective/emotional empathy: The ability or capacity to recognise emotions that are being experienced by another person, when you feel the feelings of another person along with the other person, as though their emotions are your own. Social neuroscience has found that this kind of empathy has to do with the mirror neuron system. Emotional empathy contributes to an individual being well attuned to another person's inner emotional world, an advantage for individuals in a wide range of careers from nursing to teaching to social work, psychology and other caring professions.

Compassionate empathy, or 'empathic concern': This kind of empathy helps us to understand a person's predicament and feel with them, and also be spontaneously moved to help them, if and when others need help. Under stress, theory of mind skills may appear to be completely absent.

19. Some commonly observed 'co-existing disorders' or conditions

Ehlers-danlos syndrome/hypermobility syndrome.

Irlen syndrome.

Irritable Bowel syndrome.

Adrenal gland fatigue.

Chronic fatigue syndrome.

Anxiety, stress and/or anger. Recent brain scanning research points towards amygdala's role in intense emotions, anxiety and anger.

Auditory processing issues.

Obsessive Compulsive Disorder (OCD) or traits.

One or more of the seven types of ADHD (see http://www.amenclinics.com).

Executive function difficulty (i.e. time management, planning ahead, organisation).

Sensitivities to medications, caffeine and/or alcohol.

Gluten, wheat, casein or other food allergies/intolerances, gut issues.

www.aspiengirl.com © Tania A. Marshall

19. Some commonly observed 'co-existing disorders' or conditions

Sleep difficulties or sleep disorder, a preference for staying up late at night, usually not a morning person, may keep 'vampire' hours.

May have tics (e.g. throat-clearing, coughing, and sniffing).

Epilepsy.

Learning difficulties and/or disability.

Personality disorder.

*No one woman will have all of these traits. Some of the traits in this list may not apply to you. A level of insight and awareness is required in terms of recognising the traits, characteristics and behaviours in oneself. There is high heterogeneity within the group.

**Asperger Syndrome often co-occurs with other conditions and disorders, e.g. dyslexia, dysgraphia, dyscalculia, irlen syndrome, dyspraxia/disability of written expression, auditory processing disorder and/or ehlers-danlos syndrome.

***Individuals may show varying levels of skills, talents, gifts and impairments. This is dependent on how characteristics affect the person, level of intelligence, how severe the impairment(s) is, any co-existing condition(s) and/or personality type. Individual traits and characteristics can vary from mild to severe.

APPENDIX 2
Ideas for using
I AM Aspien *Woman*

The greatest gift an AspienWoman can receive is a diagnosis. For it is through the diagnosis that she gains knowledge and understanding of herself, of where she fits in the world, and her unique profile of characteristics, strengths and challenges. It explains her experiences, both past and present, provides a starting point for her future and gives her permission to be a little easier on herself. Discussing and explaining the diagnosis in a strengths-based way is crucial to self-esteem and her future. An exploration and nurturing of talents in addition to providing tools that address her weaknesses are also important.

Professionals:

This book is a great tool to use as a visual aid to help in explaining the unique profile of strengths and challenges and the diagnosis. I recommend explaining the diagnosis in a strengths-based way. You might like to utilise the pages in the book to point out to your client some of her strengths and challenges. Working together and creating an individualised strengths/challenges profile can be very useful, to not only the client, but also to family members, co-workers, partner and/or support worker. This profile can then be utilised to assist others with understanding the client.

The majority of adults coming into a clinic or medical setting have self-diagnosed. They have spent much time questioning, researching, looking for an answer to their challenges and now would like a formal diagnosis to confirm or rule out their conclusions.

With your client, go through the pages and discuss some of the strengths first, followed by some of the weaknesses or challenges. Make two separate lists on a whiteboard or on paper. Then discuss the unique profile in its entirety, introducing the terms Autism or Asperger Syndrome and the background/history of Autism/Asperger Syndrome.

After discussing your client's unique profile, having a conversation about other successful female mentors who also have Autism or Asperger Syndrome can be a positive, hopeful and empowering next step. First, create and develop a list, including pictures, of females on the spectrum and what they have achieved or are achieving. Second, explain to your client how the individual's unique profile and strengths may have contributed to them becoming a successful musician and/or having a successful career.

Parents/Family Members/Carers:

This book can be utilised as a great visual tool for women who already have a diagnosis or those who may be self-diagnosing and now are looking for someone who works in the area to provide a formal assessment. This book can be used as an educational and/or awareness tool for family members, siblings, children, co-workers, colleagues and/or supervisors.

You:

This book can be used as a starting point in recognising your own characteristics, traits and strengths. You may have spent years trying to figure yourself out. You may have been misdiagnosed or you may be undiagnosed. You may be wondering about someone else, a loved one, family member, daughter, sister, partner. You may have read about Asperger's in males and thought that the profile didn't fit you until you read the female phenotype. You may have even read about the 'stereotypical' female Asperger's traits and felt you didn't fit in until you learned more about heterogeneity, subtypes or Broader Autism Phenotype (BAP). You can also use this book to give to your loved ones, family members, your doctor or other professionals.

APPENDIX 3
My Unique Strengths List

Developing a list of personal strengths, talents and gifts is vital to healthy self-esteem and self-identity and it is never too late to begin. Think of some qualities, personality traits, skills, talents that you like about yourself and begin your list. Ask family members, your partner, friends or co-workers what they think you are good at. Keep adding to your list on an ongoing basis. If you are having trouble thinking of any, take a look at the mentors' strengths in the previous section and see if you can identify any of those in yourself. It may be necessary to try some new things to find out if you are good at them. It's never too late to discover what your talents are.

Strength	Description
Self-Taught	For Example: Taught myself guitar and piano
Intelligence	For Example: An IQ test showed that ...
Visual Thinker	For Example: I think in pictures, moving pictures, etc., and therefore I learn best by ...
Self-Taught	
Intelligence	
Visual Thinker	
Pattern Thinker	
Word Thinker	
Sport	
Technology	
Art	
Music	
Writing	
Expertise Knowledge	
Honest	
Perfectionism	
Determination	
Intuition	
One-on-One	
Animal Empath	
Ecological Empath	
Perseverance	
Teaching	
Learning	

Add any other strengths and descriptions you can think of on this page.

Strength	Description

APPENDIX 4
20 Reasons to Obtain an Adult Formal Diagnosis

TANIA A. MARSHALL

One of the most common questions I am asked is "Should I get a diagnosis as an adult?" There are many advantages to receiving a diagnosis, at any age, and some of the more common and important advantages are as follows:

1. An explanation for feeling different.

2. Confirmation or ruling out of a self-diagnosis and co-existing conditions or disorders. Some people who self-diagnose are not on the Autism spectrum; however, many are.

3. To help and assist my child who is on the spectrum by being able to tell him/her.

4. A more appropriate label rather than thinking one is 'weird', a 'freak' or less endearing terms.

5. Awareness, self-understanding and an explanation of one's life, past or current experiences, thoughts and feelings, behaviours.

6. An awareness and understanding of family history, what other family members may have (or may have had) whether that may have been Autism or Broader Autism Phenotype (BAP).

7. Learning what kind of thinker and learner you are.

8. Receiving academic support, services and support.

9. Understanding for family members, friends, co-workers or partners.

10. An accurate diagnosis can prevent misdirected treatment (for example, medications that are not useful).

11. Prevention of future problems (e.g. individuals with Autism have a much higher suicide risk and/or can develop a personality disorder, an inappropriate work environment and/or career).

12. Helpful in understanding the best careers or jobs.

13. Learning about your own unique cognitive profile of abilities, strengths/gifts and challenges.

14. Learning your own unique sensory profile and creating and using a sensory kit and making environmental accommodations.

15. Learning the appropriate reasons for anxiety, depression, self-harm and suicidal ideation.

16. Eating disorders in Autistic people often have a different cause and need different treatment.

17. Learning how to cope in a world that is often too loud, too busy and too fast, what your triggers are, how to practise extreme self-care.

18. To learn how to communicate, recognise emotions and feelings in yourself and others.

19. Gives permission to not be so hard on yourself in regards to your challenges (e.g. "I should be more social with the other mothers. What is wrong with me?").

20. May prevent suicide (due to the increased rate of suicidal ideation and attempts in people with Autism).

Disclosure

A diagnosis does not always mean disclosure. By this, I mean disclosure may not be helpful. It depends. In my work with women, I have had women who wanted a diagnosis just for themselves and planned to tell no-one (not even their partners or family members), I have had people who have told the world, and I've had everything in between! Disclosure can have positive or negative ramifications and it is context dependent. Once you have disclosed you cannot take it back, nor can you control how or what others will say or think. In an ideal world, it would be perfect if the workplace or educational institution or other people would act according to disability law or respond how you would like them to, but this is often not the case. It may or may not benefit you to tell people and the pros and cons need to be considered, even if a workplace says they are aware and accommodating of disability.

What are the pros and cons of disclosure for you?

Be prepared that other people may not believe you

It is a common experience for women to be invalidated, disregarded and/or not believed after they disclose their diagnosis to family members, partners or friends. This is mainly due to a lack of education and/or awareness about Autistic females.

Other people may expect to see physical signs or behaviours to confirm to them that a woman is on the Autism spectrum. They may compare her to the media stereotyped characters or the males they know or know of on the spectrum. They may say inappropriate or upsetting things to the newly diagnosed, often coming from good intentions. Educating others (by referring them to research or books) and self-advocating, where possible, may be helpful.

What are some scripts or responses you can have prepared ahead of time?

Another way of talking about a diagnosis without talking about the 'A' word

Another way of discussing a diagnosis can be in the form of discussing characteristics, traits, abilities or challenges. For example, talking about neurodiversity and 'different' brains (just like there are different trees and flowers) can be a helpful analogy. Relating different trees or flowers to people gives others an understanding of different brain types. Learning to advocate for oneself is important and can be effective when done appropriately. The following are a couple of examples to get assist and reflect on.

"I'm the kind of person who likes to socialise for a little while but then I need a break to recharge my batteries."

"I'm the type of person who is really interested in talking about English literature and not so great with small talk."

"I'm an introvert and need more time alone than others so I can concentrate on my painting."

What are some ways you can explain your strengths and challenges? What are some ways you can advocate for yourself?

References

***Author's Note: The following *academic* references were either referred to and/or are helpful resources

American Psychiatric Association. (2013). *Diagnostic and statistical manual of mental disorders: DSM-5*. Washington, D.C: American Psychiatric Association.

Andersson, G., Gillberg, C., and Miniscalco, C. (2013). Pre-school children with suspected Autism spectrum disorders: Do girls and boys have the same profiles? *Research in Developmental Disabilities, 34*, 413-422.

Attwood, T. (2006). *The pattern of abilities and development of girls with Asperger's syndrome. In Asperger's and girls*. Arlington, TX: Future Horizons, Inc.

Auyeung, B., Baron-Cohen, S., Chakrabarti, B ., Lombardo, M.V., and Meng-Chuan, L. (2015). Sex/Gender Differences and Autism: Setting the Scene for Future Research. *Journal of the American Academy of Child & Adolescent Psychiatry, 54*(1): 11–24.

Banissy, M. J., and Ward, J. *Mirror-touch synaesthesia is linked with empathy*. (2007). Retrieved from http://www.daysyn. com/Banissy_Wardpublished.pdf

Baron-Cohen S, Ashwin E, Ashwin C, Tavassoli T, Chakrabarti B (2009). Talent in autism: hyper-systemizing, hyper-attention to detail and sensory hypersensitivity. *Philosophical Transactions B., 364*, 1377–1383.

Baron-Cohen, S., Jaffa, T., Davies, S., Auyeung, B., Allison, C., and Wheelwright, S. (2013). Do girls with anorexia nervosa have elevated autistic traits? *Molecular Autism, 4*, 1, 24.

Baron-Cohen, S., Lombardo, M.V., Auyeung, B., Ashwin, E., Chakrabarti, B., et al. (2011). Why are autism spectrum conditions more prevalent in males? *PLOS Biology, 9*: e1001081.

Baron-Cohen, S., Robinson, J., Wheelwright, S, Woodbury-Smith, M., ...(2007). *Very Late Diagnosis Of Asperger Syndrome*. Retrieved February 15, 2015 from http://iancommunity.org/cs/articles/very_late_diagnosis_of_ asperger_ syndrome

Begeer, S., Mandell, D., Wijnker-Holmes, B., Venderbosch, S., Rem, D., Stekelenburg, F., and Koot, H. (2012). Sex Differences in the Timing of Identification Among Children and Adults with Autism Spectrum Disorders. *Journal of Autism and Developmental Disorders, 43*, 5, 1151–1156.

Bogdashina, O. (2003). *Sensory Perceptual Issues in Autism and Asperger Syndrome: Different Sensory Experiences, Different Perceptual Worlds*. United Kingdom: Jessica Kingsley Publishers.

Bogdashina, O., and Peeters, T. (2010). *Autism and the edges of the known world sensitivities, language, and constructed reality*. United States: Jessica Kingsley Publishers.

Coombs, E., Brosnan, M., Bryant-Waugh, R., and Skevington, S. M. (2011). An investigation into the relationship between eating disorder psychopathology and autistic symptomatology in a non-clinical sample. *British Journal of Clinical Psychology, 50*, 3, 326-338.

Dworzynsky, K., Ronald, A., Bolton, P., and Happe, F. (2012). How different are girls and boys above and below the diagnostic threshold for Autism spectrum disorders? *Journal of the American Academy of Child and Adolescent Psychiatry, 51*, 8, 788-797.

Enticott, P.G., Fitzgerald, P.B., & Kirkovski, M. (2013). *A review of the role of female gender in Autism spectrum disorders. Journal of Autism and Developmental Disorders, 43*, 11, 2584-603.

Fannin, B., Nigro, J., and Orci, T. (2013, May 22). *Original Video – Bitchy Resting Face.* Retrieved from https://www.youtube.com/watch?v=3v98CPXNiSk

Frazier T. W. et al. (2014). Behavioural and cognitive characteristics of females and makes with autism in the Simons Simplex Collection. *Journal of the American Academy of Child and Adolescent Psychiatry, 53*, 329-340.

Gomez de la Cuesta, G., and Mason, J. (2010). *Asperger's Syndrome For Dummies.* John Wiley & Sons; UK Edition.

Gould, J. & Ashton-Smith, J. (2011). Missed diagnosis or misdiagnosis? Girls and women on the autism spectrum. *Good Autism Practice, 12*, 1, 34–41.

Grandin, T. and Panek, R. (2014). *The Autistic Brain: Helping Different Kinds of Minds Succeed.* Boston, MA: Mariner Books.

Halladay, A.K, Bishop., S., Constantino, J.N., Daniels, A.M., Koenig, K., Palmer, K, et. al. (2015). Sex and gender differences in autism spectrum disorder: summarizing evidence gaps and identifying emerging areas of priority. *Molecular Autism 6*, 36.

Head, A.M., McGillivray, J.A., and Stokes, M.A. (2014). Gender differences in emotionality and sociability in children with autism spectrum disorders. *Molecular Autism, 5*, 19.

Hendrickx, S. (2015). *Women and Girls with Autism Spectrum Disorder: Understanding Life Experiences from Early Childhood to Old Age.* London: Jessica Kingsley Publishers.

Hurley, E. (ed.) (2014). *Ultraviolet Voices: Stories of Women on the Autism Spectrum.* Birmingham: Autism West Midlands.

Kearns Miller, J. (2003). *Women from Another Planet?* Bloomington, IN: 1st Books Library.

Kennedy, D., Banks, R. and Grandin, T. (2011). *Bright not broken: gifted kids, ADHD, and Autism.* United Kingdom: Wiley, John & Sons, Incorporated.

Kirkovski, M., Enticott, P., & Fitzgerald, P. (2013). A review of the role of female gender in Autism spectrum disorders. *Journal of Autism and Developmental Disorders, 43*, 11, 2584-603.

Kopp, S. and Gillberg, C. (1992). Girls with social deficits and learning problems: autism, atypical Asperger Syndrome or a variant of these conditions. *European Child and Adolescent Psychiatry, 1,* 2, 89-99.

Kopp, S. and Gillberg, C. (2011). The Autism Spectrum Screening Questionnaire (ASSQ - Revised Extended Version (ASSQ-REV): an instrument for better capturing the autism phenotype in girls? A preliminary study involving 191 clinical cases and community controls. *Journal Research in Developmental Disabilities 32,* 6, 2875-88.

Lai, M.-C., Lombardo, M. V, Chakrabarti, B. and Baron-Cohen, S. (2013). Subgrouping the Autism "spectrum": reflections on DSM- 5. *PLOS Biology, 11,* e1001544.

Lai, M-C., Lombardo, M.V., Pasco, G., Ruigrok, ANV., Wheelwright, S.J., et al. (2011). A Behavioral Comparison of Male and Female Adults with High Functioning Autism Spectrum Conditions. *PLOS ONE 6,* 6, e20835.

Lai, M.-C., Lombardo, M. V., Auyeung, B., Chakrabarti, B., and Baron-Cohen, S. (2015). Sex/Gender Differences and Autism: Setting the Scene for Future Research. *Journal of the American Academy of Child and Adolescent Psychiatry, 54,* 1, 11–24.

Lai, M.C., Lombardo, M.V., Suckling, J., Ruigrok, A.N., Chakrabarti, B., Ecker, C., et al. (2013). Biological sex affects the neurobiology of autism. *Brain, 136,* 2, 799-815.

Losh, M., Adolphs, R., Poe, M.D., Couture, S., Penn. D., et al. (2009). Neuropsychological profile of Autism and the broad Autism phenotype. *Archives General Psychiatry 66,* 518–526.

Mandy, W. (2013). *DSM5 May Better Serve Girls with Autism.* New York: Simons Foundation Autism Research Initiative. Available at www.sfari.org/news-and-opinion/specials/2013/dsm-5-special-report/dsm-5-may-better-serve-girls-with-autism - Accessed on 5 March 2015

Mandy, W., Charman, T. and Skuse, D. H. (2012). Testing the construct validity of proposed criteria for DSM-5 Autism spectrum disorder. *Journal of the American Academy of Child and Adolescent Psychiatry, 51,* 41–50.

Mandy, W., Chilvers, R., Chowdhury, U., Salter, G., Seigal, A. and Skuse, D. (2012). Sex differences in autism spectrum disorder: evidence from a large sample of children and adolescents. *Journal of Autism and Developmental Disorders 42,* 7, 1304-13.

Mandy, W. and Skuse, D. (2015, March 11). *The female autism conundrum* (Webinar). In Sfari Webinar Series. Retrieved from http://sfari.org/sfari-community/community-blog/webinar-series/2015/webinar-the-female-autism-conundrum

Mandy, W. and Tchanturia, K. (2015). Do women with eating disorders who have social and flexibility difficulties really have autism? A case series. *Molecular Autism,* 6:6

Marshall, T.A. (2014). *I Am AspienGirl: The Unique Characteristics, Traits and Gifts of Females on the Autism Spectrum.* Publisher: Author

Marshall, T.A. *AspienWomen: Adult women with Asperger Syndrome. Moving towards a female profile of Asperger Syndrome.* Available at https://taniaannmarshall.wordpress.com/2013/03/26/moving-towards-a-female-profile-the-unique-characteristics-abilities-and-talents-of-asperwomen-adult-women-with-asperger-syndrome/ - Accessed on March

Nichols, S., Moravcik, G.M. and Tetenbaum, S.P. (2009). *Girls Growing up on the Autism Spectrum.* London: Jessica Kingsley Publishers.

Nordahl, C.W., Losif, A.M, Young, G.S., Perry, L.M., Dougherty R, Lee A, et.al. (2015). Sex differences in the corpus callosum in preschool-aged children with autism spectrum disorder, *Molecular Autism, 6,* 26.

Nyden, A., Hjelmquist, E. and Gilberg, C. (2000). Autism spectrum and attention deficit disorders in girls: some neuropsychological aspects. *European Child and Adolescent Psychiatry 9,* 3, 180-5.

Oldershaw, A., Treasure, J., Hambrook, D., Tchanturia, K. and Schmidt, U. (2011). Is anorexia nervosa a version of autism spectrum disorders? *European Eating Disorders Review 19,* 6, 462-74.

Shamay-Tsoory, S. G., and Tibi-Elhanany, Y. (2011). Social cognition in social anxiety: first evidence for increased empathic abilities. *The Israel journal of psychiatry and related sciences, 48,* 2, 98-106.

Solomon, M., Miller, M., Taylor, S.L., Hinshaw, S.P. and Carter, C.S. (2012). Autism symptoms and internalizing psychopathology in girls and boys with autism spectrum disorders. *Journal of Autism and Developmental Disorders, 42,* 48–59.

Takei, A., Mera, K., Sato, Y. and Haraoka, Y. (2011). High-functioning autistic disorder with Ehlers-Danlos syndrome. *Psychiatry and Clinical Neurosciences, 65:* 605–606.

University of Cambridge. (2013). *Autism Affects Different Parts of the Brain in Women and Men.* Cambridge: University of Cambridge. Available at www.cam.ac.uk/research/news/autism-affects-different-parts-of-the-brain-in-women-and-men. Accessed on 22 March, 2015.

Wijngaarden-Cremers, P.M., Eeten, E., Groen, W., Deurzen, P., Oosterling, I. and Gaag, R. (2013). Gender and age differences in the core triad of impairments in Autism spectrum disorders: a systematic review and meta-analysis. *Journal of Autism and Developmental Disorders, 44,* 1-9.

Wolff S. and McGuire, RJ. (1995). Schizoid personality in girls: a follow-up study–what are the links with Asperger's syndrome? *Journal of Child Psychology and Psychiatry, 36,* 5, 793–81.

Wylie, P. (2014). *Very Late Diagnosis of Asperger Syndrome.* London: Jessica Kingsley Publishers.

Highly Recommended Resources

AUTISM IN PINK

www.autisminpink.net

- ebook *Breaking the silence* (contains the personal stories of some of the women who took part in the project, research reports, presentations from the project's International conference and study trip to Brussels to meet MEPs and other project outputs)

- Watch the 35-minute *Autism In Pink* documentary available on YouTube

FREE WEBINAR: THE FEMALE AUTISM CONUNDRUM

featuring Dr Will Mandy and Dr David Skuse

http://sfari.org/sfari-community/community-blog/webinar-series/2015/webinar-the-female-autism-conundrum

- Learn more about the gender bias in autism

MIRROR TOUCH SYNAESTHESIA

http://www.daysyn.com/

PROFESSIONALS DIRECTORY

For more information regarding professionals around the world who work with females go to: http://taniamarshall.com/female-asc-professionals.html

Further Projects

The AspienGirl® and AspienWoman Mentor Project and Interview Series was created due to the lack of information about successful females on the spectrum and their innate strengths. Tania has been privileged to meet females of all ages with a stunning array of AspienPowers (gifts, talents, strengths and/or abilities) who are true warriors, heroines and superheroes. These females have all overcome challenges and continue to shine a light for themselves and others through their positivity and mentorship. This is what makes them a warrior.

Tania's interviews of females on the spectrum are available at www.aspiengirl.com/blog

You will find a variety of ages from a variety of places in the world who are excellent role models, mentors, heroines and superheroes, who have unique talents and strengths, and who provide inspiration and hope to others on the spectrum.

If you or someone you know would like to be a mentor for others by showcasing your talents, success or abilities, or would like to share your story in one of her books, please contact Tania at tania@aspiengirl.com

The **AspienGirl® Project** was created to address several issues:

Awareness: Females who have Autism or Asperger's are often misdiagnosed and receiving inappropriate interventions.

Advocacy: Females are marginalised members of society. AspienGirls form a minority subculture within this larger marginalised group of females and as such have unique needs and challenges.

Education: There is little knowledge of AspienGirls around the world. An important step is to make available resources about the female profile across the lifespan, gender differences, interventions and support for females, in as many languages and countries as possible. The AspienGirl® Project has donated 300 copies of *I Am AspienGirl®* to professionals, schools and organisations.

Philanthropy: AspienGirls seeking a diagnosis are often not able to afford the cost. The AspienGirl® Project will donate a percentage of book sales to cover the costs of diagnoses for those that cannot afford it.

The Be Your Own Superhero (BYOSH) Project was created to showcase females on the spectrum, of all ages, their abilities, talents, gifts and superpowers. The BYOSH Project provides an empowering, positive and strengths-based movement for females on the spectrum. #beyourownsuperhero encourages all females on the spectrum to find out what their unique strengths, talents, gifts and interests are, to foster and nurture them and to be involved in them as often as possible, for it is not whether they 'fit in' or feel the same as everyone else that should define who they are, their self-esteem or their identity.

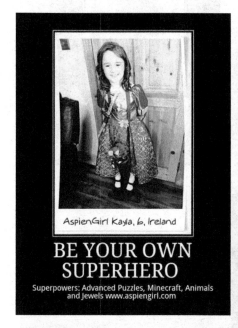

AspienGirl Kayla, 6, Ireland

BE YOUR OWN SUPERHERO

Superpowers: Advanced Puzzles, Minecraft, Animals and Jewels www.aspiengirl.com

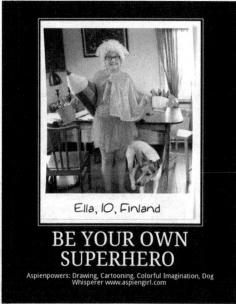

Ella, 10, Finland

BE YOUR OWN SUPERHERO

Aspienpowers: Drawing, Cartooning, Colorful Imagination, Dog Whisperer www.aspiengirl.com

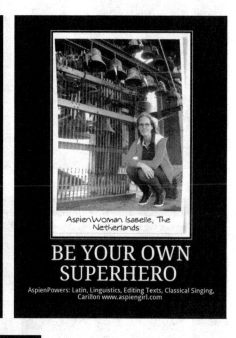

AspienWoman Isabelle, The Netherlands

BE YOUR OWN SUPERHERO

AspienPowers: Latin, Linguistics, Editing Texts, Classical Singing, Carillon www.aspiengirl.com

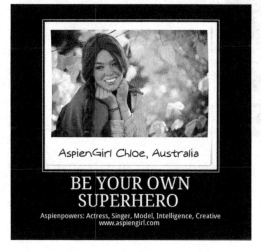

AspienGirl Chloe, Australia

BE YOUR OWN SUPERHERO

Aspienpowers: Actress, Singer, Model, Intelligence, Creative www.aspiengirl.com

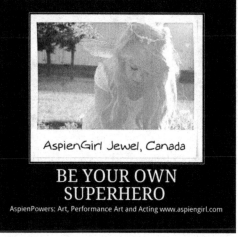

AspienGirl Jewel, Canada

BE YOUR OWN SUPERHERO

AspienPowers: Art, Performance Art and Acting www.aspiengirl.com

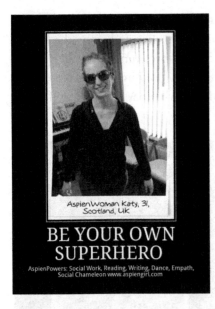

AspienWoman Katy, 31,
Scotland, UK

BE YOUR OWN SUPERHERO

AspienPowers: Social Work, Reading, Writing, Dance, Empath,
Social Chameleon www.aspiengirl.com

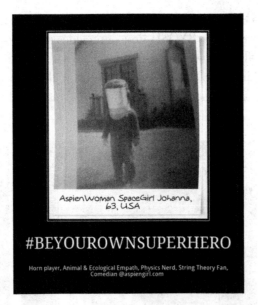

AspienWoman SpaceGirl Johanna,
63, USA

#BEYOUROWNSUPERHERO

Horn player, Animal & Ecological Empath, Physics Nerd, String Theory Fan,
Comedian @aspiengirl.com

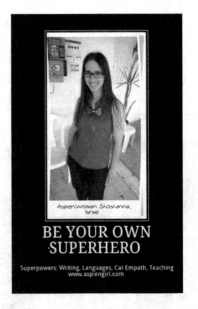

AspienWoman Shoshanna,
Israel

BE YOUR OWN SUPERHERO

Superpowers: Writing, Languages, Cat Empath, Teaching
www.aspiengirl.com

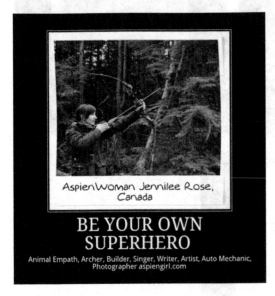

AspienWoman Jennilee Rose,
Canada

BE YOUR OWN SUPERHERO

Animal Empath, Archer, Builder, Singer, Writer, Artist, Auto Mechanic,
Photographer aspiengirl.com

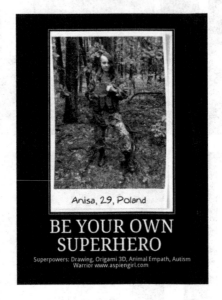

Anisa, 29, Poland

BE YOUR OWN SUPERHERO

Superpowers: Drawing, Origami 3D, Animal Empath, Autism
Warrior www.aspiengirl.com

If you would like to be a part of this project please send in your details (name, age, country you live, your superpowers and contact details) to tania@aspiengirl.com with 'Be Your Own SuperHero Project' in the subject heading.

The Planet Aspien SmartPhone App is available in both iOS and Android at https://itunes.apple.com/au/app/planet-aspien/id927392689?mt=8

Tania's female Autism app called **Planet Aspien** includes an audio section where you can listen to her radio show interviews (Autism Show, Vancouver, Canada and Positively Autistic UK), read her blog and three developmental female autism screening tools, check out the 'Be Your Own Superhero (BYOSH) Project' heroes, her social media, updates, recommended meditations, sample chapters of her books, her two websites and testimonials.

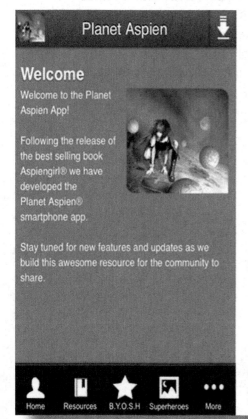
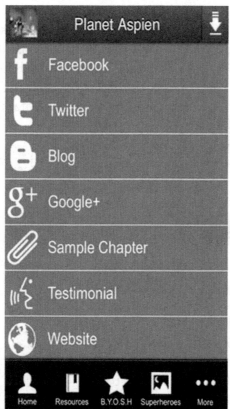
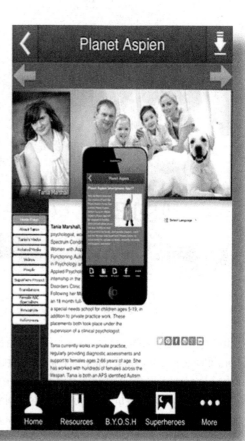

Future Titles

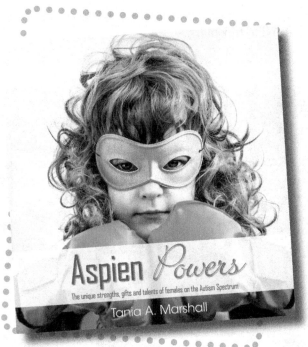

Using positive strengths-based language, Tania Marshall showcases the gifts and talents of the many females that she has personally worked with. If you have been searching for a book that describes what AspienGirls can DO, can ACCOMPLISH, and can BE, then this is the book for you. This book provides hope for any AspienGirl's future, by discussing and focusing on the unique combination of talents, strengths and gifts commonly seen in individuals with Asperger Syndrome or Autism. This book is focused on what this remarkable group of females can do and the positive future they can have, once environmental accommodations are made, strengths are identified and the focus becomes on their strengths.

Using positive strengths-based language, Tania Marshall showcases the unique profile of characteristics, traits, gifts and talents of the many young males that she has personally worked with. If you have been searching for a book that describes the variance in what young male Aspiens can DO, can ACCOMPLISH, and can BE, then this is the book for you. Whilst addressing the struggles common to twice-exceptional boys, this provides hope for any AspienBoy's future, by discussing and focusing on the unique combination of talents, strengths and gifts commonly seen in individuals with Asperger Syndrome or Autism.

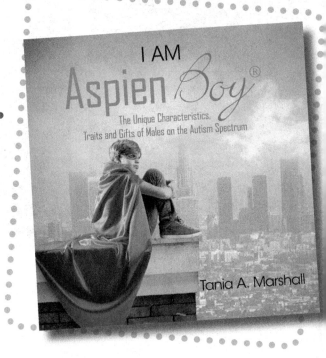

Future Titles

Behind The Mask: A Guide for Professionals Working with Females on the Autism Spectrum (2016)

This book shares the common narrative themes drawn from a large group of females, all with a diagnosis of Autism Spectrum Condition (ASC), who discuss their thoughts, experiences and feelings from their earliest memories until their present day, a span of many years.

Using a combination of research, autobiographical narratives, clinical and anecdotal observations, Tania Marshall sheds light on an often misunderstood group of females, why they are missed and/or misdiagnosed, the coping strategies and techniques used, how they hide their Autism (including the varying ways this is done), what to look for in an assessment, and what questions to ask. She discusses the kinds of environmental accommodations, helpful therapist characteristics and therapist modifications that are useful in professional practice.

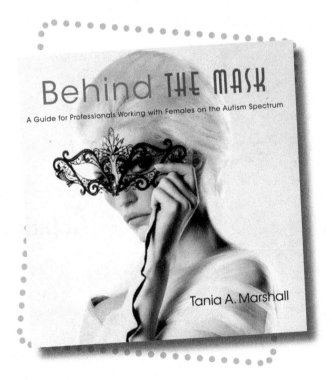

Future Titles

Author's books

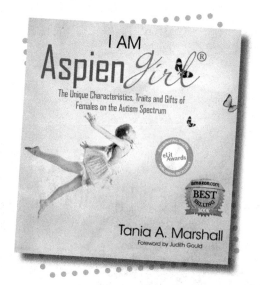

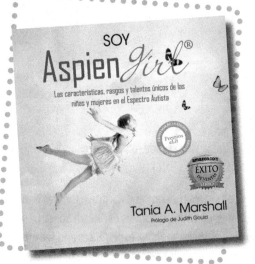

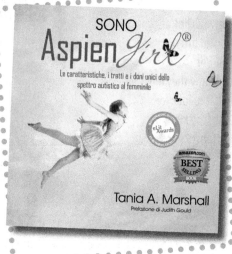

I Am AspienGirl® is being released in the following languages: Italian, Japanese, Hebrew, Dutch, Norwegian, French, Brazilian Portuguese, Danish, German and Chinese. If you would like to translate this book please email Tania at tania@aspiengirl.com

About the Author

Tania Marshall is a best-selling author and a psychologist. In 2015, she was nominated for a 2015 ASPECT Autism Australia National Recognition Award (Advancement Category) for advancing the field of female Autism and received a 2015 eLIT Gold Medal Award for her first self-published book entitled *I Am AspienGirl: The Unique Characteristics, Traits and Strengths of Females on the Autism Spectrum*, foreword by Dr Judith Gould. Tania is currently working on several books and projects and her work has been translated and/or cited in numerous publications including Sarah Hendrickx's recent release entitled *Women and Girls with an Autism Spectrum Disorder* (2015), foreword by Dr Judith Gould. Tania is trained and experienced in the field of child and family psychology, neurodiversity, Autism, Asperger Syndrome and related conditions, giftedness, Twice-Exceptional, Genius, Savant Syndrome and highly sensitive individuals. She has a Masters of Science degree in Applied Psychology and currently divides her time between private practice (diagnostic assessments, post-diagnosis support, intervention, problem-solving), writing and research.

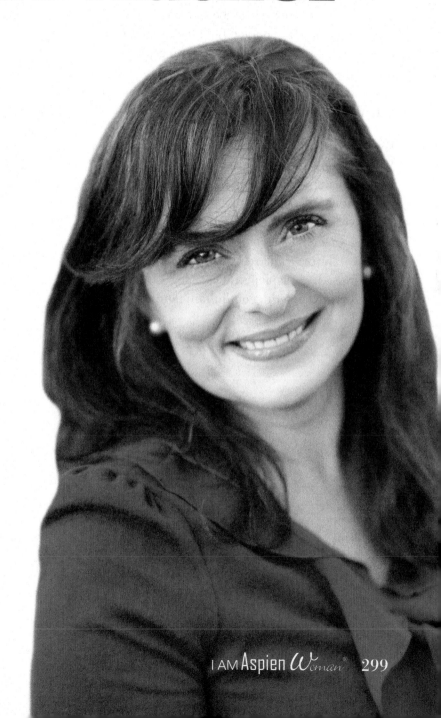

At www.aspiengirl.com you can sign up for our newsletter to stay up to date with the book series, projects, The AspienGirl® Project Webinar Series, receive free chapters of the books, tips, resources, blogs and more. To contact Tania for assessments, workshops, presentations, book signings, translating her books or for in-person or remote Skype consulting or conferencing, please email her at tania@aspiengirl.com

For more information:
W: www.aspiengirl.com
T: www.twitter.com/TaniaAMarshall
T: www.twitter.com/aspiengirlVIP
FB: www.facebook.com/taniamarshallauthor
FB: www.facebook.com/aspiengirl
Pinterest: https://pinterest.com/taniaamarshall
Wordpress: www.aspiengirl.com/blog
LinkedIn: au.linkedin.com/in/taniaannmarshall/

Notes

CPSIA information can be obtained
at www.ICGtesting.com
Printed in the USA
FSOW04n1645170417
33231FS